NEOADJUVANT CHEMOTHERAPY - INCREASING RELEVANCE IN CANCER MANAGEMENT

Edited by **Maurie M. Markman**

Neoadjuvant Chemotherapy - Increasing Relevance in Cancer Management
http://dx.doi.org/10.5772/56655
Edited by Maurie M. Markman

Contributors

Vladimir Semiglazov, Katia Hiromoto Koga, Sonia Marta Moriguchi, Gilberto Uemura, José Ricardo Rodrigues, Eduardo Carvalho Pessoa, Angelo Gustavo Matthes, Dilma Morita, Suebwong Chuthapisith, Suthinee Ithimakin, Jasmeet Singh, Amy Tiersten, Jong-Sup Park, Sung-Jong Lee, Maurie Markman

Published by InTech

Janeza Trdine 9, 51000 Rijeka, Croatia

Publishing Process Manager Ana Pantar
Technical Editor InTech DTP team
Cover InTech Design team

Additional hard copies can be obtained from orders@intechopen.com

Neoadjuvant Chemotherapy - Increasing Relevance in Cancer Management, Edited by Maurie M. Markman
p. cm.
ISBN 978-953-51-1139-9

For EU product safety concerns:
IN TECH d.o.o., Prolaz Marije Krucifikse Kozulić 3, 51000 Rijeka, Croatia,
info@intechopen.com or visit our website at intechopen.com.

Meet the editor

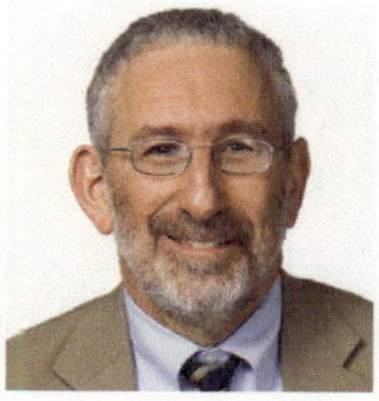

Dr. Maurie Markman is Senior Vice President for Clinical Affairs and National Director for Medical Oncology at Cancer Treatment Centers of America. He is also a Clinical Professor of Medicine at the Drexel University College of Medicine. Dr. Markman's clinical and research interests are in the area of gynecologic malignancies and specifically the development of novel treatment strategies for ovarian cancer. Prior to joining Cancer Treatment Centers of America in 2010, Dr. Markman served as Vice President for Clinical Research at the MD Anderson Cancer Center in Houston, Texas.

Contents

Preface

Neoadjuvant chemotherapy is not a new concept in cancer management. It has long been recognized that a subgroup of patients with advanced local (e.g., breast cancer) or regional (e.g., ovarian cancer) malignant disease would not be able to undergo definitive treatment to control the primary lesion. *By delivering chemotherapy first* it was hoped local control would subsequently be able to be accomplished.

A second category of patients felt to be candidates for a neoadjuvant treatment approach included individuals with significant co-morbid medical conditions (e.g., cardiac history) where it was believed to not be possible to undertake the extensive surgery required to control the local disease process due to the severity of the underlying non-malignant illness.

For example, there is a relatively a long history of the primary administration of chemotherapy to patients with extensive ovarian cancer where the surgeon felt the extent of the surgery would be problematic in view of an individual patient's baseline cardiac status. However, assuming an excellent response to chemotherapy, with an accompanying reduction in ascites and pleural effusions, surgery was felt to be able to be successfully and safely undertaken in many such patients.

However, over the past decade there has been increasing evidence that not only is neoadjuvant chemotherapy an option in some patients with extensive local or regional disease, or where an individual patient's medical status prevents a primary surgical approach, but in some settings it has become the *preferred option* based on the results of solid evidence-based phase 3 randomized trials.

The general justification for employing a primary neoadjuvant chemotherapeutic approach in several malignancies include: (a) the availability of highly biologically and clinically active anti-neoplastic agents; (b) the presence of significant volume local or regional disease making definitive local control difficult if not impossible in the absence of a substantial reduction in the tumor volume; (c) and the desire to minimize the extent of surgery while not reducing the opportunity for the most favorable survival outcome for the individual patient.

In the chapters of this excellent text, the authors have described advances in the neoadjuvant chemotherapeutic management of a number of tumor types. Based on the extensive experience with this management concept in breast cancer, several chapters are devoted to this important topic (Section 1). Section 2 deals with the administration of neoadjuvant chemotherapy in non-breast malignancies.

Those who read and study the content of the chapters that follow will come away with a far greater understanding of the rationale supporting neoadjuvant chemotherapy, the existing evidence-based data regarding its use, limitations of the approach, and required future investigative efforts to learn how to optimize the benefits of this innovative management concept.

Maurie Markman, M.D.
Senior Vice President for Clinical Affairs, Cancer Treatment Centers of America
Clinical Professor of Medicine, Drexel University College of Medicine, USA

Section 1

Neoadjuvant Chemotherapy of Breast Cancer

Chapter 1

Neoadjuvant (Preoperative) Therapy in Breast Cancer

Vladimir F. Semiglazov and Vladislav V. Semiglazov

Additional information is available at the end of the chapter

http://dx.doi.org/10.5772/53122

1. Introduction

Locally advanced breast cancer (LABC) occurs at presentation in approximately 20-25% of breast cancer patients worldwide, but significantly less in countries with implemented screening programs. LABC refers to large operable (stage IIB, IIIA) or inoperable (stage IIIB, IIIC) tumors, including inflammatory breast cancer. Patients with ipsilateral supraclavicular lymph node involvement previously considered as having metastatic disease are now also included in the category of LABC (stage IIIC). Treatment of LABC has evolved within recent decades. For a long time, mastectomy remained the mainstay of treatment in this group of patients, but long-term local control was disappointingly low, with approximately 50% local recurrences (LR) and only 2% 5-year overall survival (OS). Implementation of postoperative radiotherapy increased local control and survival, but long-term outcomes remained unsatisfactory (35-55% LR and 25-45% five-year OS). Incorporating systemic therapy (be it chemotherapy, hormonal therapy or both) as an adjunct to surgery and/or radiotherapy further improved results. Currently, a combination of systemic therapy with locoregional treatment (surgery and/or radiotherapy) constitutes the standard of care in LABC patients since improving locoregional control is associated with better survival. In patients with stage III breast cancer treated with induction chemotherapy followed by surgery, radiotherapy or a combination thereof, the risk of loco regional recurrence is in the range of 20%. The use of induction systemic therapy results in tumor downstaging, and in selected LABC patients even allows for breast conserving surgery (BCS). However, the safety and efficacy of this approach in LABC have not been verified in randomized studies. Even though locoregional management is an important component of multimodality treatment in patients with LABC, the pattern of local management and factors influencing local treatment strategy in this group are not well recognized (Sinacki et al., 2011). Neoadjuvant therapy is recommended not only for locally advanced and inflammatory breast cancer but also as an option for primary operable disease without compromising long-term outcome (Untch et al., 2011).

2. Neoadjuvant systemic therapy

2.1. Neoadjuvant chemotherapy

Patients presenting with locally advanced primary breast cancer (LAPC) are a heterogeneous group with variable outcomes with regard to local recurrence rates and survival. There is no standard or international agreement on the definition of this type of breast cancer, but one commonly used clinical staging includes patients with large primary tumours greater than 5 cm (T3) or with fixed skin or chest involvement (T4), and/or fixed axillary (N2) or ipsilateral internal mammary lymph node involvement (Mathew et al., 2008). According to TNM staging system proposed by the American Joint Committee on Cancer (AJCC), all of stage III disease is therefore considered locally advanced, as is a subset of stage IIB (T3N0). In addition, inflammatory breast cancer (T4d), with its distinct clinical presentation and worse prognosis, is included within the scope of locally advanced disease. Although the TNM system is not as widely used in some countries, it is generally accepted that locally advanced breast cancers represent those cancers that are difficult to resect with primary surgery either because of their size or extension to chest wall or skin or involvement of regional axillary lymph nodes. Compared to patients with operable primary breast cancer, patients with LAPC are at significantly higher risk of local recurrence and distant metastases and have a worse overall survival; UK figures show that patients with stage II disease have a 10-year survival rate of just under 60%, whereas this is approximately 30% for patients with stage III disease (Mathew et al., 2008).

With the widespread use of breast cancer screening, breast cancers are increasingly being diagnosed at an earlier stage. Because of this, patients with locally advanced breast cancer are less commonly seen than before. Nevertheless, there remains a group of patients who either because they do not seek advice earlier or because the tumour is more aggressive, present with locally advanced disease. Data from the American National Cancer Institute's Surveillance, Epidemiology, and End Results (SEER) program show that 7% of all breast cancer patients have stage III disease at diagnosis, although this percentage is less than 5% in the screening population. Despite this, patients with LAPC still present a significant clinical problem and exemplify a subgroup of patients where a multidisciplinary approach is particularly important to outcome.

Initially, an aggressive single modality, local therapy approach, was commonly advocated for the treatment of patients with LAPC, either in the form of radical surgery or radiotherapy. This often provided temporary local control, although on follow-up of these patients, the morbidity and recurrence rates were high and survival poor. Multimodal approach is now an established option in most patients with LAPC, especially oestrogen receptor (ER) negative tumours or aggressive ER positive tumours (e.g. some inflammatory cancers). This includes the combination of surgery and radiotherapy for local control and systemic therapy, usually chemotherapy +/ - hormone therapy. For others, such as those with strongly hormone receptor positive tumours, local treatments (i.e. surgery +/- radiotherapy) plus endocrine therapy or even primary endocrine therapy may be appropriate options. This may for example be the case in many elderly patients, some of who are medically unfit for surgery.

A large number of studies have assessed the use of neoadjuvant chemotherapy in operable primary breast cancer. Although the results in operable breast cancers suggest that the breast conserving rates can be increased, survival is no different when compared to post-operative adjuvant chemotherapy. However, patients with LAPC often have inoperable disease at diagnosis and the main goal of neoadjuvant treatment is to achieve resectability, either in the form of standard mastectomy or breast-conserving surgery. Furthermore, the clinical and histological response to neoadjuvant chemotherapy has been shown to be important predictors of recurrence and survival in studies of operable breast cancer. Neoadjuvant chemotherapy (NACT) in operable invasive breast cancer (OIBC) has been shown to increase breast conservation surgery (BCS) (Cebrecos et al., 2010). However, chemoresistant and multi focal tumours still require a mastectomy. As a consequence, today global management of these patients may include a breast reconstruction (Monrigal et al., 2011)

2.2. Definition and impact of pathologic complete response on prognosis after neoadjuvant therapy

Neoadjuvant chemotherapy represents an option for patients with early breast cancer when an indication for chemotherapy is given. Phathologic complete response (pCR) has predicted long-term outcome in several neoadjuvant studies and is therefore a potential surrogate marker for survival. However, selected trials comparing different neoadjuvant regimens have failed to demonstrate an association between pCR rate and improved outcome (von Minckwitz et al., 2012)

Methodologic limitations are likely to be the reason for this unexpected discrepancy. First, no standardized definition for pCR exists. Some trials have applied the pCR definition to the breast tumor only, whereas others have included the axillary nodes. Furthermore, some studies have included the presence of focal invasive cancer or noninvasive cancer residuals in their pCR definition whereas others have defined pCR as the complete eradication of all invasive and noninvasive cancer. Second, incidence and prognostic impact of pCR vary among breast cancer-intrinsic subtypes. For example, although patients with luminal A breast cancer show a low pCR rate, their overall prognosis is favorable, whereas patients with triple-negative (TN) breasi cancer show a high pCR rate but have an unfavorable outcome (von Minckwitz et al., 2012). Including all intrinsic subtypes might therefore attenuate the prognostic information of pCR.

Pathologic complete response (pCR) defined as no invasive and no in situ residuals in breast and nodes can best discriminate between patients with favorable and unfavorable outcomes. Patients with noninvasive or focal-invasive residues or involved lymph nodes should not be considered as having achieved pCR. pCR is a suitable surrogate end point for patients with luminal B/HER2-negative, HER2-positive (nonluminal), and triple-negative disease but not for those with luminal B/HER2-positive or luminal A tumors (von Minckwitz et al., 2012).

This is, to the best of our knowledge, the first individual patient- based pooled analysis analyzing different pCR definitions for their prognostic impact on survival of patients with breast cancer treated with neoadjuvant anthracycline-taxane-based chemotherapy. The large patient collective included sufficient subpopulations with small residual disease volume (eg, noninvasive residuals only, focal-invasive disease < 5 mm, or no invasive tumor in the breast but involved lymph nodes). Over the last decades, these subpopulations have frequently been considered to have achieved pCR. However, (von Minckwitz et al., 2012) show that these subpopulations have an increased risk of relapse and sometimes of death as well compared with the group of patients with stage ypT0 ypN0 breast cancer. pCR restricted to this stage showed the lowest adjusted HR for DFS and OS compared with the other definitions (Schott et al., 2012; von Minckwitz et al., 2012) further demonsfrate that in subgroups considered to have slowly proliferating tumors, pCR is not associated with prognosis, whereas in subgroups with highly proliferating tumors, pCR can discriminate between patients with good and poor prognosis accurately. The recently proposed clinicopathologic definition of the St Gallen panel nicely recognizes these subgroups. In fact, prognostic impact of pCR is highest in HER2-positive (nonluminal) and TN tumors, where patients achieving pCR show a prognosis comparable to that of patients with luminal A tumors.

Surprisingly, pCR was not prognostic in the luminal B/HER2positive subgroup irrespective of trastuzumab treatment. In this subgroup, pCR rates were low, despite concomitant anti-HER2 therapies, but similar outcomes were observed in the adjuvant trastuzumab studies.

In the research setting, Schott and Hayes (2012) recommend that neoadjuvant trials that are testing classic cytotoxic drugs with pCR as the primary end point should enroll only patients with ER-negative or highly proliferative tumors, given that these are the patients for whom pCR is shown to have prognostic value. In these instances, every body adoption of a uniform definition of pCR, which is substantially clarified by the data from von Minckwitz et al (2012). Uniform definitions for concepts such as pathologic complete response (pCP) can provide a framework for reporting clinical trial results in a coherent manner.

2.3. Neoadjuvant endocrine therapy

Duration of neoadjuvant hormonal treatment for breast cancer in most studies was 3-6 months. The few studies that investigated prolonged treatment with neoadjuvant endocrine therapy suggest that a further reduction in tumour size can be achieved and that even surgery can be withheld for elderly women on continuing hormonal treatment. However, the optimum duration of neoadjuvant endocrine therapy has to be established. For many years, primary systemic (neoadjuvant) therapy has been given before local treatment for women with locally advanced breast cancer in an effort to make such disease operable. Chemotherapy has been the mainstay of this approach, but more recently neoadjuvant endocrine therapy has emerged as an attractive alternative in post-menopausal women with large hormone receptor positive breast cancers. A number of randomized trials (like P024, IMPACT, PROACT) have compared various aromatase inhibitors directly with tamoxifen. An important endpoint in each of these studies has been the rate at which breast conservation has been achieved. The presence of steroid hormone receptors (ER and/or PR) are target for endocrine therapy. Preoperative chemotherapy may be less effective in postmenopausal patients with ER-positive and/or PR-positive tumors at least with respect to doxorubicin-containing or taxane-containing regimens. Pathological complete response (pCR) rates after chemotherapy were significantly higher among patients with tumors that were both ER-negative and PR-negative compared with patients whose tumors had any (even low) expression of steroid hormone receptors (Colleoni et al. 2004, 2008). In the ECTO I trial, pCR after neoadjuvant chemotherapy was observed in 42% of women with ER22 negative tumors, compared with 12% in the ER-positive group (Gianni et al. 2009). In the NSABP B-27 study, ER-negative tumors had higher rates of pCR than ER-positive tumors when treated with neoadjuvant AC, as well as when treated with AC followed by docetaxel (Bear et al., 2006). Before our trial there were few, if any, direct comparisons of primary neoadjuvant endocrine therapy with primary neoadjuvant chemotherapy in patients with hormone-responsive breast cancer.

This was an open-label, randomized phase 2 trial of once-daily endocrine therapy (exemestane or anastrozole) or chemotherapy (doxorubicin and paclitaxel, every 3 week for 4 cycles) in postmenopausal women with primary ER-positive breast cancer. A total of 239 patients with ER-positive and/or PgR-positive breast cancer (T2N1-2, T3N0-1, T4N0M0) were randomly assigned to receive neoadjuvant endocrine therapy (ET) [anastrazole 1 mg/day or exemestane 25 mg/day for 3 months, 121 patients] or chemotherapy (CT) [doxorubicin 60 mg/m2 with paclitaxel 200 mg/m2, four 3-week cycles, 118 patients]. All patients were considered to be ineligible for breast-conserving surgery (BCS) at enrollment. After BCS all patients received radiotherapy (50 Gy in 25 fractions). The median follow-up time was 5.6 years.

The primary efficacy end point was already reported (Semiglazov et al., 2007). Overall response (OR=CR+PR) was similar in the endocrine therapy group (65.5%) compared with chemotherapy group (63.6%; p>0.5). Interim analysis of this trial showed similar objective response in patients who were receiving exemestane and in patients who were receiving anastrazole. It allowed us to review and to analyze dates on all patients who were receiving aromatase inhibitors in the endocrine therapy group. There was a trend toward higher overall rates of OR and breast-conserving surgery among patients with tumors expressing high levels of ER (Allred score ≥6) in the endocrine therapy compared with the chemotherapy group (43% vs 24%, p=0.054).

After completing neoadjuvant treatment, 31 patients (13%) did not undergo surgical resection: 12.3% of patients who were receiving endocrine therapy and 13.5% of patients who were receiving chemotherapy. Twenty-two patients did not receive surgery because of disease progression. These patients were switched to the other study therapy: patients initially treated with endocrine therapy received chemotherapy, and patients treated with chemotherapy received endocrine therapy. Progressive disease was observed in 9% of patients who were receiving endocrine therapy and 9% of patients who were receiving chemotherapy (P>0.5). Stable disease was seen in 21% of patients who were receiving endocrine treatment and 26% of patients who were receiving chemotherapy.

Analysis of BCS rates according to pretreatment characteristics showed a non-significant trend towards increased BCS in patients with clinical stage T2, ER+/PgR+, 70 years and older (p=0.054- 0.088) receiving neoadjuvant endocrine therapy.

The rate of BCS was particularly marked in patients receiving endocrine therapy, who achieved a clinical response. There was no significant difference between endocrine therapy

(ET) and chemotherapy (CT) relative to the incidence of locoregional recurrences and distant metastases (8.2% and 7.6%, p=0.99; 14.8% and 15.2%, p=0.83, respectively). There was no significant difference in DFS through 5 years of follow up between the 121 patients who received neoadjuvant endocrine therapy and 118 women who received chemotherapy: 71.0% and 67.7% (p>0.5). After a median follow up of 5.6 years 35 events had been reported in the endocrine group (24 in 66 patients who underwent mastectomy and 11 in 40 patients who underwent BCS). 5-year DFS was 63.6% after mastectomy and 72.5% after BCS (p=0.076). The incidence of commonly reported adverse events was higher in patients receiving chemotherapy. No serious adverse events were reported in patients receiving endocrine therapy. Six patients receiving chemotherapy experienced febrile neutropenia leading to treatment interruption. No deaths occurred during the preoperative therapy. Our trial has shown that preoperartive endocrine therapy with aromatase inhibitors offers the same rate of overall objective response, breast-conserving surgery, 5-years DFS as chemotherapy in postmenopausal patients with ER-positive tumors. The frequency of adverse events was higher among patients who were receiving chemotherapy. Endocrine treatment was well tolerated. Preoperative endocrine therapy with aromatase inhibitors is a reasonable alternative to preoperative chemotherapy for postmenopausal women with ER35 positive disease in clinical situation in which the low toxicity of the regimen is considered an advantage. According St.Gallen recommendation (Goldhirsch et al., 2009) neoadjuvant endocrine therapy without chemotherapy was considered reasonable for postmenopausal patients with strongly receptor-positive disease. If used, such treatment should be considered for a duration of 5-8 months or until maximum tumour response.

2.4. Neoadjuvant therapy in HER2+ breast cancer

Amplification or overexpression, or both, of human epidermal growth factor receptor-2 (HER2, also known as ERBB2), a transmembrane receptor tyrosine kinase, is present in around 22% of early breast cancers, 35% of locally advanced and metastatic tumours, and 40% of inflammatory breast cancers, and is associated with aggressive disease and poor prognosis (Ross et al., 2009). Patients with HER2-positive locally advanced or inflammatory breast cancer are therefore in particular need of effective treatment. Trastuzumab (Herceptin, Roche, Basel, Switzerland), a recombinant humanized monoclonal antibody that targets HER2, has efficacy as monotherapy (Baselga et al., 2005) and improves results of chemotherapy in patients with HER2-positive metastatic (Slamon et al., 2001; Marty et al., 2005) and early operable breast cancer (Smith et al., 2007; Romond et al., 2005; Slamon et al., 2005). It is widely approved for use as monotherapy and in combination with chemotherapy or hormone therapy in these patients, but not specifically in those with locally advanced or inflammatory breast cancer. In a pilot study, anthracycline and paclitaxel were successfully combined with trastuzumab in patients with metastastic disease (Bianchi et al., 2003). To reduce the risk of cardiac toxic effects, only three cycles of doxorubicin were given in the pilot study, which corresponds to a cumulative dose of 180 mg per m2 of body surface area (Gianni et al., 2009). No patient developed symptomatic cardiac dysfunction, although four patients (of 16) had reversible asymptomatic decreases in left ventricular ejection fraction to 50% or lower.

The neoadjuvant Herceptin (NOAH) study was designed to assess efficacy of neoadjuvant chemotherapy with trastuzumab followed by adjuvant trastuzumab versus neoadjuvant chemotherapy alone in patients with HER2-positive locally advanced or inflammatory breast cancer. The NOAH study randomized 228 patients with centrally confirmed HER2+ locally advanced breast cancer to a chemotherapy regimen consisting of 3 cycles of doxorubicin plus paclitaxel (AT); 4 cycles of paclitaxel (T); and 3 cycles of cyclophosphamide, methotrexate, and fluorouracil (CMF), with and without trastuzumab. The addition of trastuzumab significantly improved overall response rate (81% vs 73%, P =0. 18) and pCR rates (43% vs 23%, P =0,002) (Gianni et al., 2010).

The primary objective was to compare event-free survival, which was defined as time from randomization to disease recurrence or progression (local, regional, distant, or contralateral) or death from any cause, in patients with HER2-positive disease treated with and without trastuzumab.

Trastuzumab significantly improved event-free survival in patients with HER2-positive breast cancer (3-year event-free survival 71% [95% CI 61-78; n=36 events] with trastuzumab, vs 56% [46-65; n-51 events] without; hazard ratio 0.59 [95% CI 0-38-0-90]; p-0.013). Trastuzumab was well tolerated and, despite concurrent administration with doxorubicin, only two patients (2%) developed symptomatic cardiac failure. Both responded to cardiac drugs. The results of the NOAH study have shown that in patients with HER2-positive locally advanced or inflammatory breast cancer, addition of 1 year of trastuzumab (starting as neoadjuvant and continuing as adjuvant therapy) to neoadjuvant chemotherapy improved overall response rates, almost doubled rates of pathological complete response, and reduced risk of relapse, progression, or death compared with patients who did not receive trastuzumab. Investigators recorded a benefit of trastuzumab in all 1 subgroups tested,including women with inflammatory disease (27% of HER2- positive patients) who benefited substantially from trastuzumab (Baselga et al., 2005; Semiglazov et al., 2011)

The results of the NOAH study consolidate those of other studies of trastuzumab in the neoadjuvant setting. In these mainly non-randomised studies, pathological complete response rates (variously defined) ranged from 17% to 73%, and were better than they were in historical' or concurrent HER2-negative controls (Gluck et al., 2008; Untch et al., 2008). One randomised trial in patients with operable non-inflammatory disease was stopped early when the pathological complete response rate in the trastuzumab group was more than twice as high as that of the control group (65% vs 26%) (Buzdar et al., 2005). Patient numbers in this study were small, but preliminary results from another randomized study also show a doubling in pathological complete response rate in the trastuzumab group. These response rates to primary systemic therapy are a surrogate for relapse-free and overall survival in patients who were unselected for HER2 status.

Despite concurrent use of doxorubicin, paclitaxel, and trastuzumab in the NOAH trial, incidence of symptomatic cardiac failure was low (<2%) and less than was expected (2.8- 4.1%) on the basis of adjuvant trials in which trastuzumab was given concurrently with paclitaxel after completion of doxorubicin and when trastuzumab was given as monotherapy after completion of a range of cytotoxic regimens (2%). These findings support the accumulating evidence that trastuzumab can be given concurrently with anthracyclines with a low frequency of symptomatic cardiac dysfunction, provided that low cumulative doses or less cardiotoxic anthracyclines are used, and careful cardiac monitoring is done.

The addition of trastuzumab to neoadjuvant sequential anthracycline-taxane chemotherapy (with and without capecitabine) was also investigated in the phase III GeparQuattro study, and led to a doubling of pCR rates (31.8% vs 15.4%, P <0.001) (Von Minckwitz et al., 2008). With the emergence of lapatinib (Tykerb), a dual tyrosine kinase inhibitor against HER1 and HER2, the CALGB is conducting a randomized phase III trial to evaluate paclitaxel with trastuzumab or lapatinib, or both in the preoperative setting. Several other trials are ongoing to evaluate these 2 drugs in the neoadjuvant setting, including Neo-ALTTO (Neoadjuvant Lapatinib and/or Trastuzumab Treatment Optimization) in phase III and CHERLOB in phase II.

Trastuzumab (H) in combination with chemotherapy improves outcomes in patients with HER2-positive breast cancer and is integral to the standards of care for these patients. However, in some patients disease progression still occurs. Pertuzumab (P) and trastuzumab (H) target different epitopes of HER2, and their use in combination has demonstrated improvement in response rates. NEOSPHERE study (Gianni et al., 2011) assessed the efficacy and safety of pertuzumab added to trastuzumab-based neoadjuvant chemotherapy in women with HER2-positive operable, locally advanced/inflammatory breast cancer who had not received prior cancer therapy.

Patients (n = 417) with HER2-positive (IHC3+ or IHC2+ and FISH/CISH+) breast cancer were randomized 1:1:1:1 to receive 4 neoadjuvant cycles of docetaxel (T) plus H, THP, HP or TP. Pertuzumab (P) was given at a loading dose of 840 mg and 420 mg maintenance, trastuzumab (H) at a loading dose of 8mg/kg and 6 mg/kg maintenance, and docetaxel (T) at 75 mg/m2 with escalation to 100 mg/m2 if tolerated in a 3weekly schedule. The primary endpoint was pCR in the breast.

About 40% of patients had locally advanced/inflammatory breast cancer and approximately 50% were ER/PR negative. THP combination (docetaxel + trastuzumab + pertuzumab) significantly improved the pCR rate compared with TH (docetaxel + trastuzumab) alone: 45.8% (95% CI 36.1-55.7) vs 29.0% (95% CI 20.6-38.5), P = 0.0141. Patients receiving THP (docetaxel + trastuzumab + pertuzumab) had the highest pCR rate regardless of ER/PR status, although the greatest treatment benefit in all 4 arms was observed in ER/PR-neg patients. The chemotherapy-free HP (trastuzumab+pertuzumab) arm achieved a pCR rate of 16.8%. THP (docetaxel + trastuzumab + pertuzumab) had a similar safety profile to TH. The incidence of AEs was lowest in the HP (trastuzumab+pertuzumab) arm.

Thus, the addition of pertuzumab to trastuzumab-based neoadjuvant chemotherapy resulted in a significant improvement of the pCR rate with no new safety signals of concern. Pertuzumab and trastuzumab have complementary mechanisms of action as pertuzumab inhibits HER2:HER3 heterodimerisation, thereby providing a potential mechanism to overcome tumour escape. These results support the rationale for a planned Phase III, double-blind, placebo-controlled trial evaluating pertuzumab added to standard trastuzumab-based therapy it women with HER2- positive breast cancer.

Dual HER2 inhibition is being examined in neoadjuvant and adjuvant settings. The Neo-ALTTO (Neoadjuvant Lapatimib and/or Trastuzumab Treatment Optimisation) study showed that the addition of lapatinib plus trastuzumab to neoadjuvant chemotherapy resulted in a higher pathologic complete response rate compared with the addition of trastuzumab or lapatimib monotherapy (51.3% v 29.5% v 24.7%, respectively; P<.01). Also objective (clinical) response rates at 6 weeks with anti-HER2 therapy alone were 67.1%, 30.2%, and 52.6%, respectively; those at surgery after 18 weeks of neoadjuvant anti-HER2 therapy plus chemotherapy were 80.3%, 70.5%, and 74.0%, respectively, suggesting that the combination is beneficial in the neoadjuvant setting (Baselga et al., 2012; Blackwell et al 2010-2012).

Despite the dramatic improvement in the outcome of HER2+ breast cancers since the widespread use of HER2-directed therapies, such as trastuzumab, patients continue to develop recurrences and disease progression. The mechanisms of intrinsic and acquired resistance to trastuzumab are likely multifactorial and are being exploited by the use of novel targeted agents in clinical development. The phosphoinositide-3-kinase (PI3K) pathway plays a key role in resistance to trastuzumab through increased signaling through upstream growth factor receptors, PTEN mutations, and other mechanisms, and therefore, is an excellent target for drug development in patients with trastuzumab-resistant, HER2+ breast cancers. Available clinical trials demonstrate encouraging activity of mTOR inhibitors in combination with trastuzumab monotherapy or trastuzumab-based chemotherapy in patients with HER2+ metastatic breast cancer pretreated with trastuzumab with or without lapatinib. The results of early-stage clinical trials are currently being confirmed in 2 large phase III trials (Brachman et al, 2009; Vazguez-Martin et al, 2009). Other agents, targeting the PI3K pathway, are in early clinical development for HER2+ breast cancers.

2.5. Triple-negative breast cancer

Triple-negative (ER-negative, PgR-negative, and HER2 receptor-negative) breast cancers (TNBC) account for approximately 15% of all breast cancers and, though in and of itself it is a heterogeneous group, it often exhibits an aggressive phenotype with a generally poor prognosis. Unlike HER2+ or hormone receptor- positive breast cancers, triple-negative tumors lack an established therapeutic target and though initially responsive to many standard treatment regimens, progression and recurrence can be rapid and refractory to alternative approaches. Loss or inactivation of breast cancer type 1 (BRCA1) leads to defects in certain DNA repair pathways. Most BRCA1 mutant breast cancers lack ER, PgR, and HER2 expression, and this association has raised the question of defective BRCA1 function in sporadic (non-familial) TNBC (Sorlie et al., 2003). This led to the hypothesis that triple-negative tumors may be more sensitive to DNA damaging agents, such as platinums. A retrospective analyses of patients with triple-negative breast cancer who received taxane/platinum-based primary chemotherapy demonstrated an overall response of 39% (Uhm et al., 2009), while studies of platinum monotherapy or combinations in the neoadjuvant setting have produced pCR rates of 22%-50% (Garber et al., 2006; Chang et al., 2008; Byrski et al., 2009; Schott et al., 2011).

3. Molecular profiling in prognosis and patient selection for neoadjuvant systemic therapy

Gene expression profiling with the use of DNA microarrays has added valuable information to our understanding of breast cancer biology. In the seminal work of Perou et al. (2011) the ability to interrogate thousands of genes at the same time was translated into a "molecular portrait" of each tumor sample studied, and the concomitant analysis of the individual molecular portraits of breast cancer tumor samples made the definition of molecular subtypes of breast cancer possible (Perou et al., 2011). In order to analyze this large quantity of information (thousands of genes per sample evaluated), a hierarchical clustering method was used to group genes according to similar patterns of expression. The proposed molecular classification of breast cancer was divided into five classes: luminal-A, luminal-B, basal-like, HER2-positive and normal-like tumors (Sotiriou et al., 2003; Sorlie et al., 2003). Subsequently, the correlation between molecular subtypes and clinical data have shown a significant difference in overall survival between the subtypes.

Despite this progress, the clinical applicability of molecular classification is limited by the tight correlation between the molecular subtypes and currently available immunohistochemical markers (ER, PR, HER2, Ki67) (Sotiriou & Pusztai, 2009). For example, the molecular subtype HER2-positive is clinically detected by IHC or fluorescent in situ hybridization (FISH) according to published guidelines (Sauter et al., 2009). Although a good correlation has been established between the molecular subtype HER2 and clinically assessed HER2-positive breast cancer, the opposite is not true, because 30% of HER2-positive breast cancers are molecularly characterized as luminal-B (Cheang et al., 2009). Luminal-A and luminal-B molecular subtypes are, by definition, hormone receptor positive tumors, but the distinction between these two subtypes is controversial.

One of the proposed clinical definitions characterizes luminal-A and luminal-B tumors using hormone receptor status, HER2 status and the Ki67 index (percentage of Ki67-positive nuclei by IHC). Luminal-A is defined as being ER- and/or PR-positive, HER2-negative and Ki67-low (Ki67 index < 14%). Luminal-B is defined as ER- and/or PR- positive, HER2- negative and Ki67-high (Ki67 index > 14%). Another luminal-B subtype has also been proposed, namely luminal HER2 enriched, with tumors being ER- and/or PR- positive, HER2-positive and Ki67-high (ki67 index > 14%) (Perou, 2011).

Study Jinno et al (2011) was to evaluate the clinical utility of breast cancer intrinsic subtypes in the prediction of pathological complete response (pCR) in a cohort of breast cancer patients receiving neoadjuvant chemotherapy.

Patients with stage II/III breast cancer received 4 cycles of chemotherapy XT (capecitabine 1650mg/m2 on days 1-14 and docetaxel 60mg/m on day 8 every 3 weeks), followed by 4 cycles of FEC (fluorouracil 500 mg/m2, epirubicin 90mg/m2, cyclophosphamide 500mg/m2). Immunohistochemical (IHC) analysis of ER, PgR, HER2. EGFR, cito-ceratine 5/6. and Ki67 was performed in core needle biopsy samples at baseline. Tumors were classified as luminal A (ER+ and/or PgR+, and Ki67<20%), Luminal B (ER+ and PgR+, and Ki67 > 20%). Luminal-HER2 (ER+ and/or PgR+, and HER2+), HER2-enriched (ER- PgR-, and HER2+), or triple-negative (ER-, PgR-, and HER2-). Triple-negative tumors with and without EGFR+ and/or cito-ceratine 5/6+ were further classified as basal-like and non-basal-like TN (NBTN), respectively. Pathologic complete response (pCR) was defined as no microscopic evidence of residual viable tumor cells, invasive or noninvasive, in all resected specimens of the breast. Twenty-six (31.3%) patients were classified as luminal A, 12 (14.5%) were luminal B, 15 (18.1%) were luminal-HER2, 9 (10.8%) were HER2, 10 (12.0%) were basal like, and 11 (13.3%) were NBTN. The overall response rate was 90.4%, including a complete response in 30 patients and a partial response in 45 patients. The overall pCR rate was 15.5% (12/83). The highest pCR rate (40.0%) was observed in patients with basal- like tumors. In triple-negative patients, basal-like patients showed significantly higher pCR rate than NBTN patients (40.0% vs. 9.1%. p = 0.01). There were no cases with pCR in a cohort of luminal HER2 subtype patients. A higher proportion of luminal B patients had 1 pCR than luminal A patients (25.0% vs. 3.8%, p = 0.01). Data indicate that breast cancer subtypes are useful predictive biomarkers of pCR in breast cancer patients treated with neoadjuvant systemic chemotherapy.

According Sanpaolo et al (2011) study, breast cancer subtype seems a prognostic factor of breast cancer specific survival and distant metastases rates, but not of local relapse rate. Patient could be submitted to conservative surgery, if feasible, but considering the differenced in survivals, patients with worse prognosis should receive more aggressive adjuvant treatment.

The goals of neoadjuvant therapy of breast cancer have significantly changed and evolved since it was firstly applied to women with inoperable locally advanced and inflammatory breast cancers in the early 1970's. The extended indication to allow more breast conserving surgery has widened the application of neoadjuvant treatments and provided evidence for the association between favorable long term outcome and intermediate endpoints, like pathologic complete response (pCR) after chemotherapy or decreased tumor proliferation measured by Ki87 after endocrine therapy. A key question is whether pCR and Ki87 can take the role of qualified and validated surrogate markers of drug efficacy, so that any difference in survival between treatments disappeared after adjustment for the intermediate endpoint. The recent improvements in understanding the molecular basis of breast cancer heterogeneity has provided a new level of complexity but also an outstanding conceptual framework for interpreting the role of' pCR as potential surrogate marker, and has made clear that the biologic meaning of pCR is different in different molecular subtypes, and that different molecular subtypes will require different intermediate surrogate endpoints. The validation of the intermediate surrogates markers of efficacy would dramatically change the landscape of development of new drugs for early breast cancer and do provide the rationale for a comparative analysis of the intermediate endpoint instead of the final survival endpoint. The feasibility of this major paradigm shift from large and lengthy adjuvant clinical trials to smaller and faster neoadjuvant trials is still the topic of discussion, and will be addressed by regulators, biostatisticians, translational scientists and oncologists.

4. The surgical aspects of neoadjuvant therapy

4.1. The surgical management of patient who achieve a complete pathological response after neoadjuvant therapy

Neoadjuvant systemic treatment (NST) is the standard treatment for locally advanced breast cancer (BC) and a standard option for primary operable disease. This analysis aimed to identify whether breast cancer patients receiving radiotherapy alone following a complete clinical remission (cCR) to neoadjuvant chemotherapy had a worse outcome than those treated with surgery.

We identified 8 studies of NST where breast cancer patients who achieved a cCR were eligible for different types of local management: radiotherapy only or surgery. Primary outcomes were loco-regional recurrence, distant disease free survival (DDFS), overall survival (OS) (Semiglazov, 2008; Clouth et al., 2007; Ring et al., 2004; Smith et al., 2002).

We performed subgroup mefa-analyses for the primary outcomes on the basis of local management. Heterogeneity between the risk ratios for the same outcome between different studies was assessed by use of the chi-square-based Q statistic.

Rates of pathologic complete response (pCR) range from 25% to 35,8% of patients who had a cCR. If a cCR is considered as a "test" of pCR then the positive predictive value of cCR in all eligible trials was low (range from 29.9% to 35%). For surgery and no surgery (radiotherapy alone) groups respectively there were no significant differences in DDFS (summary risk ratio [RR]=0.94, 95% confidence interval [CI]=0.91- 1.07) or OS (RR= 1.00, 95% CI=0.99- 1.12). But there was trend towards increased loco-regional recurrences for the radiotherapy only group (difference in favor to surgery range from 11% to 20%; RR= 1.53, 95% CI= 1.11- 2.10; P=O.02).

In patients achieving a cCR to neoadjuvant chemotherapy, radiotherapy alone achieve survival rate as good as with surgery, but with higher local recurrence rate. A prospective randomized trial addressing the need for surgery after cCR would seem reasonable in patient with magnetic resonance or positron emission tomography-defined complete remissions.

4.2. Role of sentinel node biopsy after neoadjuvant systemic therapy

The surgical management of patients presenting early stage breast cancer (T1- T2) and clinically negative lymph nodes (NO) has long included both primary tumor resection and level I/II axillary lymph node dissection (ALND). This last procedure has been largely substituted by the sentinel lymph node biopsy (SLNB) which is nowadays recommended by most clinical guidelines for this subgroup of patients. Indeed, the well documented accuracy of SLNB in predicting the axillary status implies that, in these patients, a negative sentinel lymph

http://dx.doi.org/10.5772/53122

node (SLN) is considered sufficient to rule out metastases in other axillary nodes and to avoid axillary dissection. Several randomized clinical trials have further indicated that SLNB and ALND are comparable in terms of overall survival and incidence of nodal failure (Canavese et al., 2011).

Over the years, neo-adjuvant chemotherapy (NAC) has become the preferred treatment for patients with operable locally advanced breast cancer, in an attempt to reduce the tumor mass and to favor breast-conservative surgery over mastectomy. In addition, NAC has been shown to down-stage the axillary status in some 30-40% of the patients treated. Based on the SLNB validation studies mentioned above, it would be reasonably legitimate to introduce the SLNB procedure also in the context of NAC. However, one frequent adverse effect of NAC is the anatomical alteration of the lymphatic drainage, with lymphatic vessels disrupted by tumor, inflammation or fibrosis, or blocked by necrotic and/or apoptotic cells; in addition, NAC could induce a non-uniform tumor regression in the axillary nodes, being most effective in some nodes but not in others.

These events could prevent a proper diffusion of the scintigraphic tracer during lymphatic mapping, in the one hand, and contribute to a reduction in the rate of successful SLN identification and, more importantly, an increase in the rate of false-negative SLN. Therefore, the demonstration of the feasibility and accuracy of SLNB after NAC is of major interest since in the future responders to NAC who would be down-staged to a negative nodal status (NO) could be spared a complete axillary dissection and the immediate sequelae of axillary surgery. Two large NSABP trials have incorporated SLN biopsy either before chemotherapy (B-32, 5536 patients) or after NAC (B-27, 428 patients) and report comparable mapping success (97% vs 89%) and false negative rates (9.8% vs 9.3%) for combined blue dye and radioactivity.

There is a current SNB trial looking at SNB before and after neoadjuvant systemic therapy in Germany called SENTINA(Kuehn et al., 2009). This is a four arm study. Patients who are clinically node-negative have SLNB prior to NAC. Those who are SLNB negative at diagnosis have no further axillary procedure after NAC whereas those who are SLNB

Positive proceed after NAC to a further SLNB and axillary dissection. Clinical node-positive patients have primary systemic therapy and those that are clinically node-negative go on to have SLNB and axillary lymph node dissection, whereas those who are clinically node-positive undergo axillary lymph node dissection alone. Over 600 patients have been enrolled to date. The study design is somewhat complex but will add to the body of knowledge on the value of ALNB after NAC

Dixon and Cody (2010) recommend that all patients at diagnosis have axillary ultrasound and that any suspicious nodes should be submitted to fine needle aspiration cytology or core biopsy. Those who appear to be node-negative on the basis of clinical exam, imaging, and needle biopsy should have SLN biopsy post-NAC, at the same time as their breast surgery, to assess the extent of any remaining disease. Those with proven axillary node metastases at diagnosis should also be considered for SLN biopsy post-NAC. For patients with triple-negative or HER2-positive disease there is a more than 50% chance that all involved nodes will be sterilized by NAC +/- trastuzumab. This contrasts to patients with ER-positive disease who have an approximate 4% rate of axillary node sterilization. These data can be used to inform patients at the outset of treatment as to the possible surgical options for the axilla after NAC. For patients with involved nodes at diagnosis who have a complete clinical and imaging response in the axilla, SLN biopsy is reasonable post-NAC and ALND can be avoided if the SLN is negative. For the remaining patients whose nodes remain positive post-NAC (less than half of those with triple-negative or HER2-positive cancers, and over 95% of those with ER-positive disease), ALND should remain the standard of care.

So intra-operative lymphatic mapping and SLNB are nowadays part of the standard management of patients with early-stage breast cancer and clinically negative axillary nodes. Based on the present results, this procedure is feasible and is an accurate predictor of the axillary nodal status also when it is performed after NAC in patients with locally advanced breast cancer. However, before introducing SLNB as a routine procedure in the context of NAC, clinical trials will have to demonstrate that overall survival and disease-free survival do not worsen when ALND is not performed in the subset of post-NAC SLN-negative patients, thus leaving behind down-staged axillary nodes.

5. Conclusion

The neoadjuvant (preoperative, primary) use of cytotoxic, hormonal, and/or trastuzumab therapy effectively reduces tumor burden in the breast and the axilla without compromising survival. The risk of local recurrence is determined by the initial clinical stage and the pathologic stage after neoadjuvant therapy. Neoadjuvant therapy is indicated in patients with inoperable tumors or if BCT is desired by patients with large tumors otherwise requiring mastectomy. Patients with multicentric tumors generally will not become candidates for BCT with this approach. Initial multidisciplinary evaluation is important. The tumor site should be marked before treatment (eg, by clipping) to allow tumor localization at surgery. Multiple imaging studies are not needed during treatment unless there is concern about disease progression. Surgery is necessary in all patients, even those with a complete clinical response. Any residual palpable or imaging-detected lesions should be removed, but the entire initial rumor volume does not need to be resected in tumors showing a reduction in size. The optimal timing of sentinel lymph node biopsy in relation to neoadjuvant systemic therapy in patients with a clinically lymph node-negative axilla is uncertain at this time, and further study is required. The identification rate of the sentinel lymph node appears to be lower after neoadjuvant therapy, but some patients may avoid axillary lymph node dissection because of downstaging. Ultrasonography of the axilla in clinically lymph node-negative patients is useful in identifying pathologically lymph node-positive patients at presentation. In some cases, knowledge of the pretreatment lymph nodal status is useful for radiation planning. In patients with lymph node-positive disease at presentation who become clinically lymph node-negative after treatment, axillary dissection is recommended because of the high false-negative rate of SNB in this circumstance. Postoperative radiation therapy is recommended for all patients treated with breast-conserving surgery and for all patients with initially lymph node-positive disease or with locally advanced disease treated with mastectomy.

Acknowledgment

We thank Dr. J. Bryanceva For the preparation of the references.

Author details

Vladimir F. Semiglazov[1] and Vladislav V. Semiglazov[2]

1 Petrov Research Institute of Oncology, Russia

2 St.Petersbug Pavlov Capital Medical University Russia, Russia

References

[1] Baselga, J., Carbonell, X., & Castaneda-Soto, N. (2005). Phase II study of efficacy, safety, and pharmacokinetics of trastuzumab monotherapy administered on a 3-weekly schedule. J Clin Oncol, 0073-2183x, 23, 2162-2171.

[2] Baselga, J., Semiglazov, V., Van Dam, P., Manikhas, A., & Bellet, M. (2009). Phase II Randomized Study of Neoadjuvant Everolimus Plus Letrozole Compared With Placebo Plus Letrozole in Patients With Estrogen Receptor-Positive Breast Cancer. Journal of Clinical OncologyJune 1), 0073-2183x, 27(16), 2630-2637.

[3] Bianchi, G., Albanell, J., & Eiermann, W. (2003). Pilot trial of trastuzumab starting with or after the doxorubicin component of a doxorubicin plus paclitaxel regimen for women with HER2-positive advanced breast cancer. Clin. Cancer Res. 1078-0432, 9, 5944-5951.

[4] Blackwell, K. L., Burstein, H. J., & Storniolo, A. M. (2010). Randomized study of lapatinib alone or in combination with trastuzumab in women with ErbB2-positive, trastuzumab refractory metastatic breast cancer. J Clin Oncol. , 28, 1124-1130.

[5] Blackwell, K. L., Burstein, H. J., Storniolo, A. M., Rugo, H. S., Sledge, G., Aktan, G., Ellis, G., Florance, A., vukelja, S., Bischoff, J., Baselga, J., & O'Shaughnessy, J. (2013). Overall survival benefit with lapatinib in combination with trastuzumab for patients with human epidermal glowth factor receptor 2- positive metastatic breast cancer: finalresults from the EGF104900 Study. J Clin Oncol. , 30, 2585-2592.

[6] Brachmann, S., Hofmann, I., & Schnell, C. (2009). Specific apoptosis induction by the dual PI3K/mTOR inhibitor NVP-BEZ235 in HER2 amplified and PIK3CA mutant breast cancer cells. Proc Natl Acad Sci USA, 0027-8424, 106, 22299-22304.

[7] Buzdar, A., Ibrahim, N., Francis, D., Booser, D., Thomas, E., & Theriault, R. (2005). Significantly higher pathological complete remission(PCR) rate after neoadjuvant therapy with trastuzumab, paclitaxel and epirubicin chemotherapy: Results of a randomized trial in human epidermal growth factor receptor 2-positive operable breast cancer. J.Clin Oncol. 0073-2183x, 23, 3676-3685.

[8] Canavese, G., Dozin, B., Vecc, Hio. G., Tomei, D., & Villa, G. (2011). Accuracy of sentinel lymph node biopsy after neo-adjuvant chemotherapy in patients with locally advanced breast cancer and clinically positive axillary nodes. EJSO. N , 37, 688-694.

[9] Cataliotti, L., Buzdar, A., & Noguchi, S. (2006). Comparison of Anastrozole versus Tamoxifen as Preoperative Therapy in Postmenopausal Women with Hormone Receptor- Positive Breast Cancer: The Pre-operative "Arimidex" Compared to Tamoxifen (PROACT) Trial. Trial. Cancer.0000-8543x, 106(10), 2095-2103.

[10] Cebrecos, I., Cordoba, O., Deu, J., Xercavins, J., & Rubio, I. (2010). Can we predict local recurrence in breast conservative surgery after neoadjuvant chemotherapy? EJSO. N ISSN, 36, 528-534.

[11] Chang, H., Slamon, D., & Gornbein, J. (2008). Preferential pathologic complete response (Pcr) by triple-negative (-) breast cancer to neoadjuvant docetaxel (T) and carboplatin (C.). J. Clin. Oncol., suppl), abstract 604), 0073-2183x, 26, 31s.

[12] Cheang, M., Chia, S., & Voduc, D. (2009). Ki67 Index, HER2 Status, and Prognosis of Patients with luminal B Breast Cancer. J Natl Cancer Inst, 0027-8874, 101, 736-750.

[13] Clouth, B., Chandrasekharan, S., Inwang, R., Smith, S., Davidson, N., & Sauven, P. (2007). The surgical managlment of patients who achieve a complete pathological response after primary chemotherapy for locally advanced breast cancer. EJSO. ISSN, 33, 961-966.

[14] Colleoni, M., Viale, G., & Zahrieh, D. (2004). Chemotherapy is more effective in patients with breast cancer not expressing steroid hormone receptors: a study of preoperative treatment. Clin Cancer Res, 1078-0432, 10, 6622-6628.

[15] Colleoni, M., Viale, G., Zahrieh, D., Bottiglieri, L., Gelber, R., Veronesi, P., Balduzzi, A., Torrisi, R., Luini, A., Intra, M., Dellapasqua, S., Cardillo, A., Ghisini, R., Peruzzotti, G., & Goldhirsch, A. (2008). Expression of ER, RgR, HER1, HER2, and response: a study of preoperative chemotherapy. Ann. of Oncology, N.3. (March 2008), 0923-7534, 19, 465-472.

[16] Dixon, J., & Cody, H. (2010). Role of sentinel node biopsy in patients having neoadjuvant chemotherapy. EJSO. N ISSN., 36, 511-513.

[17] Eiermann, W., Paepke, S., & Appfelstaedt, J. (2001). Preoperative treatment of post-menopausal patients with letrozole: a randomized double-blind multicenter study. Ann Oncol,. 12, 1527-1532, 0923-7534.

[18] Garber, J. E., Richardson, A., & Harris, L. (2006). Neo-adjuvant cisplatin (CDDP) in "triple-negative" breast cancer (BC). Breast Breast Cancer Res TreatRes Treat suppl 1), S 149 (abstract 3074), 0167-6806, 100

[19] Gianni, L., Baselga, J., Eiermann, W., Porta, J., & Semiglazov, V. (2009). Phase III trial evaluating the addition of paclitaxel to doxorubicin followed by cyclophosphamide, metotrexate and fluorouracil as adjuvant or primary systemic therapy: European Co-operative Trial in Operable Breast Cancer. J. Clin Oncol, May 2009), 0073-2183X, 27(15), 2474-2481.

[20] Gianni, L., Eiermann, W., Semiglazov, V., Manikhas, A., & Lluch, A. (2010). Neoadjuvant chemotherapy with trastuzumab, followed by adjuvant trastuzumab versus neoadjuvant chemotherapy alone, in patients with HER-positive, locally advanced breast cancer (the NOAH trial): a randomized controlled superiority 1 trial with a parallel HER2-negative coh. ort. The Lancet0140-6736, 375, 377-384.

[21] Gianni, L., Pienkowski, T., Roman, L., Tseng, L., & Liu, M. (2011). Addition of pertuzumab(p) to trastuzumab (H)-based neoadjuvant chemotherapy significantly improves pathological complete response in women with HER2-positive early breast cancer: result of a randomized phase II study (NEOSPHERE). The Breast. suppl 1 (March 2011), 0960-9776, 20, 573.

[22] Gluck, S., Mc Kenna, E., Jr , , & Royce, M. (2008). Capecitabine plus docetaxel, with or without trastuzumab, as preoperative therapy for early breast cancer. Int J Med Sci. 1449-1907, 5, 341-346.

[23] Goldhirsch, A., Ingle, J., Gebber, R., Coates, A., Thurlimann, B., & Senn, H. (2009). Annals of Oncology, N 4 (June 2009), 0923-7534, 20, 1133-1144.

[24] Jinno, H., Matsuda, S., Sakata, M., Hayashida, T., Takahashi, M., & Hirose, S. (2011). Differential pathologic response from primary systemic chemotherapy across breast cancer intrinsic subtypes. The Breastsuppl 1. (March 2011), 0960-9776, 20, 39.

[25] Kaufman, M., Morrow, M., von, Minckwitz. G., & Harris, J. (2010). Locoregional treatment of primary breast cancer/ Cancer- January,- , 116, 1184-1191.

[26] Kuehn, T., Bauerfeind, I., Fehm, T., (2009, , & , S. E. N. (2009). SENTinel node biopsy before or after neoadjuvant systemic treatment: the German SENTINA trial. Cancer ResearchPost Presented at 32nd San Antonio Breast Cancer Conference, December 2009., 69(1008)

[27] Marty, M., Cognetti, F., & Maraninchi, D. (2005). Randomized phase II trial of the efficacy and safety of trastuzumab combined with docetaxel in patients with human epidermal growth factor receptor 2-positive metastatic breast cancer administered as first-line treatment: the M77001 study group. J. Clin.Oncol, 0073-2183x, 23, 4265-4274.

[28] Mathew, J., Asgeirsson, K., Cheung, K., Chan, S., Dahda, A., & Robertson, J. (2009). Neoadjuvant chemotherapy for locally advanced breast cancer: A review of the literature and future directions. EJSO. N 2 (February), 0748-7983, 35, 113-122.

[29] Monrigal, E., Dauplat, J., Gimbergues, P., Bouedec, G., & Reyronie, M. (2011). Mastectomy with immediate breast reconstruction after neoadjuvant chemotherapy and radiation therapy. A new option fir patients with operable invasive breast cancer. Results of a 20 years single institution study. EJSO. ISSN, 37, 864-870.

[30] Perou, C. (2011). Molecular classification of breast cancer and its emerging clinical relevance. The BreastSuppl. 1 (March 2011), 0906-9776, 20, S2-S3.

[31] Ring, A., Smith, I., & Ashley, S. (2004). Oastrogen receptor status, pathological complete response and prognosis in patients receiving neoadjuvant chemotharapy for early breast cancer. Br J Cancer, 0007-0920, 91, 2012-2017.

[32] Romond, E., Perez, E., & Bryant, J. (2005). Trastuzumab plus adjuvant chemotherapy for operable HER2-positive breast cancer. N Engl J Med, 1533-4406, 353, 1673-1684.

[33] Sapado, P., Barbieri, V., & Genovesi, D. (2011). Prognostic value of breast cancer subtypes on breast cancer specific survival, distant metastases and local relapse rates in conservatively managed early stage breast cancer: A retrospective clinical study. EJSO. ISSN., 37, 876-882.

[34] Sauter, G., Lee, J., & Bartlett, J. (2009). Guidelines for human epidermal growth factor receptor 2 testing biologic and methologic consider ations. J Clinic Oncol, 0073-2183x, 27, 1323.

[35] Schott, A., & Hayes, D. (2012). Defining the benefits of neoadjuvant chemotherapy for breast cancer. J. Clin. Oncol. ISSN, 30, 1747-1749.

[36] Schott, S., Sohn, C., Schneeweiss, A., & Heil, J. (2011). Preoperative systemic treatment in BRCA-positive breast cancer patients: case repot and review of literature. Breast Care. ISSN, 6, 395-398.

[37] Semiglazov, V., Eiermann, W., Zambetti, M., Manikhas, A., & Bozhok, A. (2011). Surgery following neoadjuvant therapy in patients with HER2-positive locally advanced or inflammatory breast cancer participating in the neoadjuvant herceptin (NOAH) study. EJSO. N ISSN, 37, 856-863.

[38] Semiglazov, V. How to handle breast cancer patients with complete response following neoadjuvant chemotherapy? ((2008). EJSO. Vol N ISSN, 1025.

[39] Semiglazov, V., Kletsel, A., & Semiglazov, V. (2005). Exemestane (E) vs tamoxifen (T) as neoadjuvant endocrine therapy for postmenopausal women with ER+ breast cancer(T2N1-2,T3N0-1,T4N0M0)[abstract]. J Clin Oncol ASCO Annual Meeting Proceedings [Post- Meeting Edition], S), 0073-2183x, 223, 530.

[40] Semiglazov, V., Semiglazov, V., Dashyan, G., Ziltsova, E., & Ivanov, V. (2007). Phase II randomized trial of primary endocrine therapy versus chemotherapy in postmeno-

pausal patients with estrogen receptor-positiv breast cancer. Cancer, 0000-8543x., 110, 244-254.

[41] Semiglazov, V., Topuzov, E., & Bavli, J. (1994). Primary(neoadjuvant) chemotherapy and radiotherapy compared with primary radiotherapy alone in stage IIb-IIIa breast cancer. Ann Oncol, 0923-7534, 5, 591-595.

[42] Semiglazov, V. F., & Semiglazov, V. V. Neoadjuvant systemic therapy in breast cancer ((2012). Chapter 1 in book "Neoadjuvant chemotherapy- current applications in clinical practice" (Edited by Oliver F.Bathe). In Tech, Rijeka, Cloatia, 978-9-53307-994-3, 1-22.

[43] Sinacki, M., Badzio, A., Welnicka-Jaskiewicz, M., Bogaerts, J., & Piccart, M. (2011). Patter of care in locally advanced breast cancer: focus on local therapy. The Breast. N ISSN, 20, 145-150.

[44] Slamon, D., & Eiermann, W. (2005). Phase III randomized trial comparing doxorubicin and cyclophophomide followed by docetoxel(FC-T) with doxorubicin and cyclophophomide followed by docetaxel and trastuzumab (AC-TH) with docetoxel,carboplatin and trastuzumab(TCH) in HER2 positive early breast cancer patients: BCIRG 006 study. Breast cancer Res Treat, suppl 1), S5, 0067-6806, 1

[45] Slamon, D., Leyland-Jones, B., & Shak, S. (2001). Use of chemotherapy plus a monoclonal antibody against HER 2 for metastatic breast cancer that over expresses HER2. N Engl J Med, 1533-4406, 344, 783-792.

[46] Smith, I. (2004). Anstrozole versus tamoxifen as preoperative therapy for oestrogen receptor positive breast cancer in postmenopausal women: Combined analysis of the IMPACT and PROACT trials. Presented at 4th European Breast cancer Conference, Hamburg, Germany.

[47] Smith, I., Dowsett, M., & Ebbs, S. (2005). Neoadjuvant treatment of postmenopausal breast cancer with anastrazole, tamoxifen, or both in combination: The immediate preoperative anastrazole, tamoxifen, or combined with tamoxifen(IMPACT) multicenter double-blind randomized trual. J Clin Oncol, N 22, 0073-2183x, 23, 5018-5116.

[48] Smith, I., Heys, S., & Hutcheon, A. (2002). Neoadjuvant chemotherapy in breast cancer: significantly enhanced response with docetaxel. J Clin Oncol., 0073-2183x, 20, 1456-1466.

[49] Smith, I., Procter, M., & Gelber, R. (2007). For the HERA study team 2 year Follow-up of trastuzumab after adjuvant chemotherapy in HER2- positive breast cancer. A randomized controlled trial. Lanset, 0140-6736, 369, 29-36.

[50] Sorlie, T., Tibshirani, R., & Parker, J. (2003). Repeated observation of breast tumor subtypes in independent gene expression data sets. Proc Natl Acad Sci USA, 0027-8424, 100, 8418-8423.

[51] Sotiriou, C., & Pusztai, L. (2009). Gene-expression signatures in breast cancer. N. Engl J Med, 1533-4406, 360, 790-800.

[52] Sotiriou, C., Neo, Sy., & Mc Shane, L. (2003). Breast cancer classification and prognosis based on gene expression profiles from a population-based study. Proc Natl Acad Sci USA, 0027-8424, 100, 10393-10398.

[53] Tutt, A., Robson, M., & Garber, J. (2009). Phase II trial of the oral PARP inhibitor olaparib in BRCA-deficient advanced breast cancer. J Clin Oncol, suppl) 803s (abstract CRA501), 0073-2183x, 27

[54] Uhm, J., Park, Y., & Yi, S. (2009). Treatment outcomes and clinicopathologic characteristics of triple-negative breast cancer patients who received platinum-containing chemotherapy. Int J Cancer, 0020-7136, 124, 1457-1462.

[55] Untch, M., Fasching, P., Konechny, G., von, koch. F., & Conrad, U. (2011). PREPARE trial: a randomized phase III trial comparing preoperative, dose-dense, dose intensified chemotherapy with epirubicin, paclitaxel and CMF versus a standard- dosed epirubicin/cyclophosphamide followed by paclitaxel +/- darbepoltin alfa in primary breast cancer- results at the time of surgery. Ann of Oncology. N ISSN, 22, 1988-1998.

[56] Untch, M., Rezai, M., & Loibl, S. (2008). Neoadjuvant treatment of HER2 overexpressing primary breast cancer with trastuzumab given concomitantly to epirubicin/cyclophosphamide followed by docetaxelcapecitabine. First analysis of efficacy and safety of the GBG/AGO multicenter intergroup-study "GeparQuattro". 6th European Breast Cancer Conference. Berlin, Germany, April Abstr 1LB, 15-19.

[57] Vazguez-Martin, A., Oliveras-Ferreros, C., & del Barco, S. (2009). m TOR inhibitors and the anti-diabetic biguanide metphormin: new insights into the molecular management of breast cancer resistance to the HER 2 tyrosine kinase inhibitor lapatinib (Tykerb). Clin Transl Oncol, 0169-9048x, 11, 455-459.

[58] Voduc, K., Cheang, M. C. U., & Tyldesley, S. (2010). Breast cancer subtypes and the risk of local and regional relapse. J Clin Oncol, 0073-2183x, 28, 1684-1691.

[59] Von, Minckiwitz. G., Rezai, M., & Loibl, S. (2008). Effect of trastuzumab on pathologic complete response rate of neoadjuvant EC-docetaxel treatment I HER overexpressing breast cancer: Results of the phase III Gepar-Qattro study (abstract 226).ASCO Breast Cancer Symposium., 2.

[60] Von, Minckwitz. G., Kummel, S., & Vogel, P. (2008). Intensified neoadjuvant chemotherapy in early- responding breast cancer: phase III randomized GeparTrio study. J Natl Cancer Inst. 0027-8874, 100, 552-562.

[61] Von, Minckwitz. G., Kummel, S., & Vogel, P. (2008). Neoadjuvant vinorelbin- capecitobine versus docetaxel-doxorubicin-cyclophosphimide in rarly nonresponsive breast cancer: phase III randomized Gepar Trio. J Natl Cancer Inst. 0027-8874, 100, 542-551.

[62] Von, Minckwitz. G., Untch, M., Blohmer-U, J., Costa, S., & eidtmann, H. (2012). Defition and impact of pathologic complete response on prognosis after neoadjuvant che-

motherapy in various intrinsic breast cancer subtypes. J Clin Oncol. N ISSN, 30, 1796-1804.

[63] Wolmark, N., Wang, J., Mamounas, E., Bryant, J., & Ficher, B. (2001). Preoperative chemotherapy in patients with operable breast cancer: nine year results from National Surgical Adjuvant Breast and Bowel Project B-18. J Natl Cancer Inst Monogr. 0027-8874, 30, 96-102.

Chapter 2

Monitoring the Response to Neoadjuvant Chemotherapy in Breast Cancer

Katia Hiromoto Koga, Sonia Marta Moriguchi,
Gilberto Uemura, José Ricardo Rodrigues,
Eduardo Carvalho Pessoa,
Angelo Gustavo Zucca Matthes and
Dilma Mariko Morita

Additional information is available at the end of the chapter

http://dx.doi.org/10.5772/53123

1. Introduction

The World Health Organization (WHO) estimates that more than 1,050,000 new cases of breast cancer occur per year worldwide, making this one of the most common diseases among women. Its mortality/incidence relationship in developed countries is 29.9%, whereas in developing countries it reaches 42.9% [1].

In developing countries, it is still a reality to find a large number of tumors in advanced stages. This is due to age [2], psychological disorders [3], racial and socioeconomic differences, besides the biological behavior of the tumor. In Brazil they are associated with the problems related to limitations in the infrastructure of the health system [4].

Data from the Surveillance Epidemiology and End Results (SEER) show between 1985 and 1995 ratios of stage III and IV tumors (advanced tumors) were respectively 18.3% (11.6% +6.7%) and 11.6% (7.4%+4.2%) [5]. On the other hand, data obtained from the registry of the Barretos Cancer Hospital, evaluated the period from 1985 to 2007, divided into four periods, showed that there was little change in the advanced tumors (III + IV), corresponding to 37.7%, 35.0%, 39.4% and 34.9% respectively, which makes the locally advanced tumors a public health problem this way.

Treatment of breast cancer is less mutilating and more effective when the diagnosis is made early. Currently, the primary systemic treatment for locally advanced tumors is advocated in order to obtain a better therapeutic response, however there is controversy in respect to this subject.

Locally advanced breast carcinoma (LABC) represent a relatively heterogeneous group, in terms of clinical, biological and pathological. Tumors locally advanced and non-metastatic involve: tumors with a diameter greater than 5 cm, large lymph node involvement (N2 or N3), direct involvement of the chest wall or skin, and inflammatory carcinoma [6].

The staging of patients with LABC suggests care, thus, those with tumors larger than 5 cm associated with more than three compromised axillary lymph nodes it is advisable that the staging be performed with computed tomography of the abdomen, thorax and pelvis, where the presence of metastatic disease, can be observed in up to 23% of cases [7]. However, its applicability in clinical routine is still a matter of controversy.

Currently, the therapeutic approach of LABC is multidisciplinary, consisting of neoadjuvant chemotherapy, surgery, radiotherapy and adjuvant chemotherapy [8-10]. In the past, the treatment of LABC was surgery, followed by chemotherapy. However, 5-year survival was less than 20%. The first reports of the application of neoadjuvant chemotherapy in LABC dating from the 70s, was initially used in inoperable patients to allow the best resection of the neoplastic lesion. In subsequent decades, with a large number of publications, an improvement was demonstrated in survival of patients undergoing this type of treatment, more evident in those with complete pathologic responses [11]. Although preclinical models suggest that neoadjuvant chemotherapy may have an impact on tumor biology and improved survival when compared to adjuvant therapy, this has not been demonstrated by clinical study in meta-analysis [12,13]. However, the primary therapy provides an *in vivo* model to evaluate the effectiveness of specific therapeutic regimen, in contrast with adjuvant therapy.

Neoadjuvant chemotherapy or primary systemic therapy suggests offering diverse advantages in relation to adjuvant, being:

- administration of medications through an intact vascular-lymphatic system;
- early treatment of micro-metastatic disease;
- *in vivo* assessment of response to treatment;
- an opportunity to evaluate the response to chemotherapy in relation to diverse clinical and pathological parameters;
- assessment of response to chemotherapy in the identification of tumor subtypes genotypic;
- reduction of tumor volume, causing in an increase in the percentage of resectability and the rate of conservative surgery;
- opportunity of evaluation of the response to new chemotherapeutic schemes;
- prior knowledge of the patient's prognosis, in function to the clinicopathologic response to chemotherapy.

http://dx.doi.org/10.5772/53123

Unfortunately, some malignant breast tumors show resistance to treatment with the principal chemotherapeutic agents, decreasing the effectiveness of this therapy [14]. The mechanisms responsible for this chemoresistance are multifactorial [15], being a late resistance acquired during treatment of predominant factor, present in over 75% of patients. The intrinsic chemoresistance is also important, being observed in 18-51% of untreated carcinomas [16-18].

In regards to chemotherapy drugs, the taxanes, have been featured in more recent studies, they showed excellent anti-neoplastic activity, then being brought to neoadjuvant chemotherapy.

The chemotherapy schemes with anthracycline and taxane combined in various ways, being concurrent or sequential demonstrate a rate of pathologic complete response (pCR) significantly higher. Based on the Aberdeen study [19] and in GEPAR-TRIO [20] the current trend is the sequential combination of anthracycline with taxane, which shows larger response rate initially obtained with anthracycline (85% vs 64%, $p = 0.03$).

The pCR is defined as the absence of invasive carcinoma in anatomopathological exam of breast and axillary lymph nodes after neoadjuvant chemotherapy. In most extensive studies, the rate of pCR ranges from 3 to 30%. However, in these same studies the criteria varies for evaluation of pCR [11].

Results showed that the long-term survival is associated to the response to neoadjuvant treatment, in patients with large volume tumors, being the pathologic complete response, the best predictor of survival in these patients [21].

Therefore, the evaluation of the response to chemotherapy treatment is important for conduct, once that the additional time and side effects triggered by this therapy are not negligible.

Reduction in tumor volume has been used as the standard criterion for response evaluation among solid tumors such as breast carcinoma. The clinical and pathological responses are used for imaging methods to define the two classifications the "World Health Organization" (WHO), created in the 70s, and the RECIST (Response Evaluation Criteria in Solid Tumors), created in the 90s [22]. The difference between the two classifications is shown in Table 1. Apparently a diameter seems to be sufficient to predict response, however the number of articles on this subject is limited.

Response	WHO	RECIST
Complete Response (CR)	Without Disease	Without Disease
Partial Response (PR)	50% response	30% Response
Stable Disease	Without PD or PR	Without PD or PR
Progression (PD)	25% increase	20% increase
Measures	2 measures	1 measure

Table 1. Difference between the classifications responses to neoadjuvant chemotherapy WHO and RECIST

2. Clinical evaluation

Feldman e cols. [23] showed significant discrepancy between chemotherapy response assessed by clinical exam and pathological study of the surgical specimen. Clinical examination is often unable to differentiate a residual mass representing fibrosis from a mass representing residual tumor [24-28].

3. Mammography

Currently the most effective imaging method for the detection of breast cancer is mammography. It has an accuracy of around 90% for mass screening. However, the extent of the tumor may be underestimated with this technique. Tabar [29] refers to practical explanations of the difficulty in assessing tumor size depending on the type and compliance of the mammary tissue represented radiologically. Similar problems to the clinical exam were observed when mammography was used for chemotherapy response evaluation [24-26]. Thus, due to difficulties in the visualization and subsequent measurement of the tumor, other imaging methods are proposed for the evaluation of chemotherapy response.

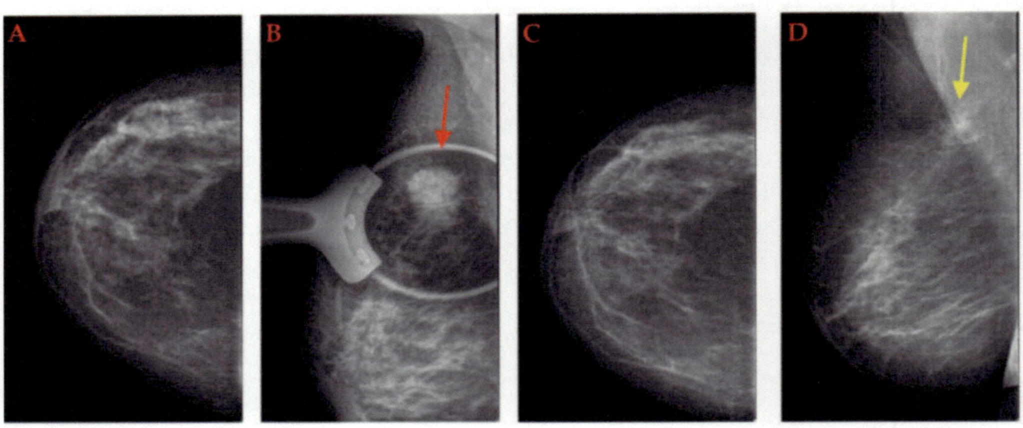

Figure 1. Mammography. Pretreatment. A. Cranial-caudal view (CC): not observed the tumor area. B. Mediolateral-oblique view (MLO) localized compression: nodular oval image, high-density, partially obscured edges with and without microcalcifications inside (red arrow). Post-treatment. C. Cranial-caudal view (CC): not observed the tumor area. D. Mediolateral-oblique view (MLO): architectural distortion in the tumor region (yellow arrow).

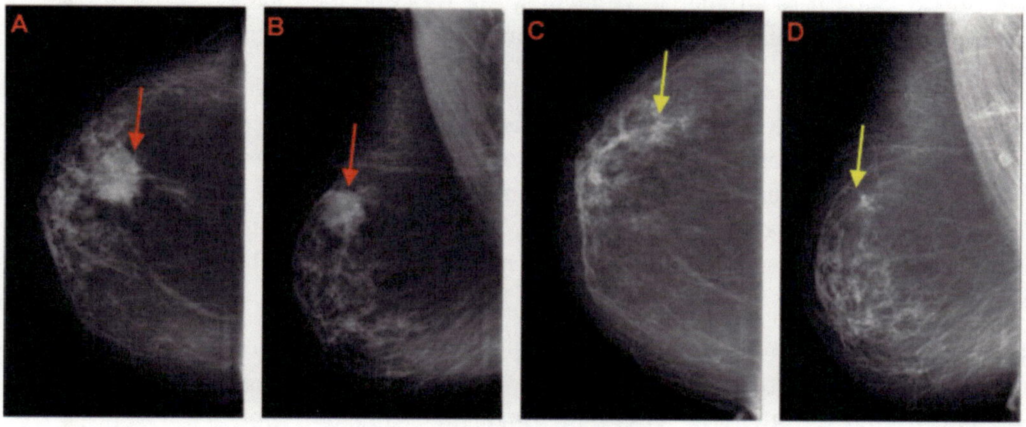

Figure 2. Mammography. Pretreatment. A. Cranial-caudal view (CC). B. Mediolateral-oblique view (MLO): area rounded nodular, spiculated margins, without microcalcifications, high density (red arrow). Post-treatment. C. Cranial-caudal view (CC). D. Mediolateral-oblique view (MLO): nodule with the same characteristics and reduction of dimensions, with partial response (yellow arrow).

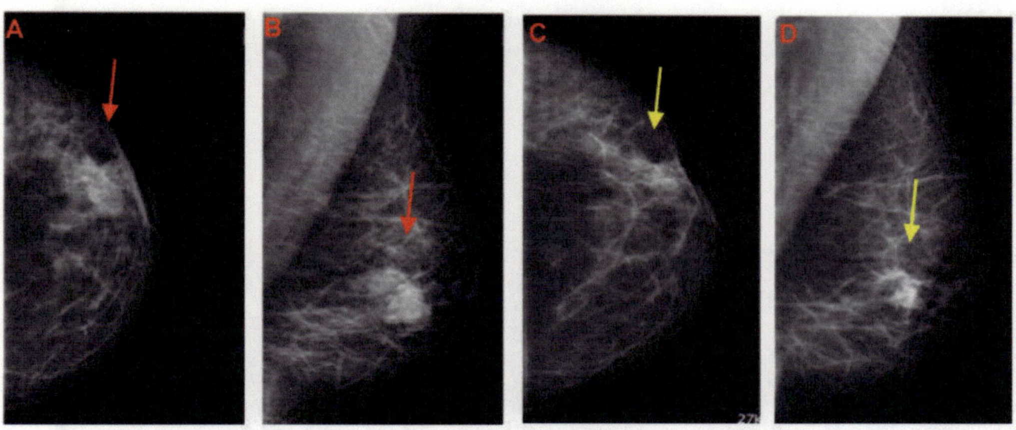

Figure 3. Mammography. Pretreatment. A. Cranial-caudal view (CC). B. Mediolateral-oblique view (MLO): rounded nodule, ill-defined margins, high density (red arrow). Post-treatment. C. Cranial-caudal view (CC). D. Mediolateral-oblique view (MLO): nodule with the same characteristics, with inadequate response (yellow arrow).

4. Breast ultrasound

Breast ultrasound is the method of choice for the determination of solid and cystic lesions. Apparently showing a more effective method in the determination of tumor measurements, however the results were not consistent. [30]

Ultrasound using it as an alternative method for assessing the tumor may predict the response to systemic treatment via the use of primary color Doppler.

Doppler ultrasound vascularization includes evaluation of parameters such as: the number of signs of flow, a peak flow velocity, the resistivity index (RI) and pulsatility index (PI). It also allows the noninvasive evaluation of abnormal vessel architecture in breast tumors, referred to as neoangiogenesis. These changes in vascularization of the tumor correlate to the histopathological response, and therefore, the study of vascularization can be used as a complementary tool to assess the response to chemotherapy, primarily in locally advanced breast cancer.

Kumar et al. [31] registered a reduction of Doppler flux during the neoadjuvant treatment in 77% of patients with partial or complete remission, the residual flux was parameter independent, having sensitivity of 88.88% for predicting pathologic complete response, compared with 44.44% clinical response.

New studies observed changes in vascularization during chemotherapy. In the beginning of chemotherapy there was an increase in vascularity, followed by a reduction thereof. Probably in the beginning of treatment, abundant angiogenic factors, such as vascular endothelial growth factor (VEGF) are released from apoptotic and necrotic tumor cells, resulting in profound increase in vascularity. After the vascularization peak, there is a gradual decrease in the later stage of chemotherapy, due to the smaller number of angiogenic factors. Thus, an increase in velocity greater than 5% was observed during chemotherapy in patients with good response to chemotherapy [32].

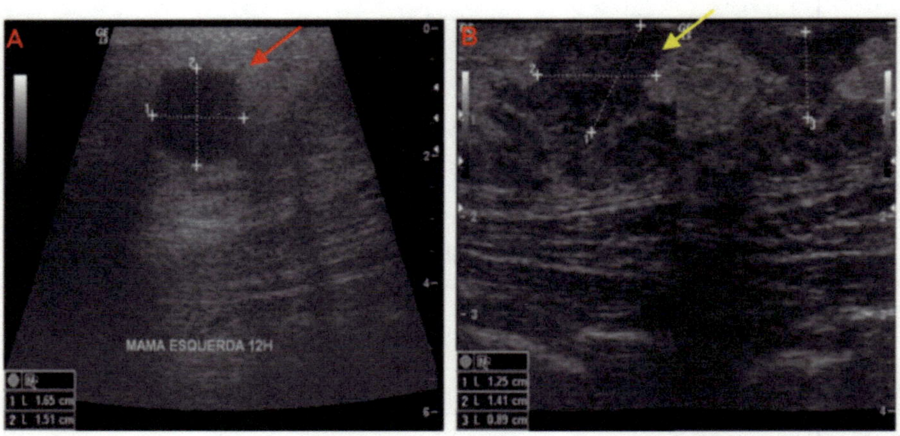

Figure 4. Breast ultrasound. A. Pretreatment: Nodule irregular, margin not circumscribed, hypoechoic, with posterior acoustic enhancement in the left breast (red arrow). B. Post-treatment: not displayed initial tumor, only nodular image of different characteristics of the initial tumor, with good response (yellow arrow).

http://dx.doi.org/10.5772/53123

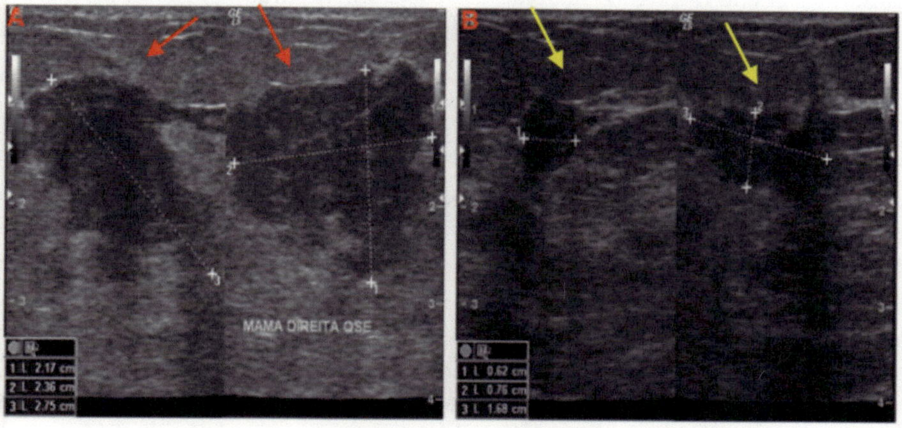

Figure 5. Breast ultrasound. A. Pretreatment: pleomorphic mass, microlobulated margins, abrupt boundary, hypoechogenic, not parallel, without posterior acoustic shadow (red arrow). Post-treatment: mass reduction pleomorphic (yellow arrow), with partial response.

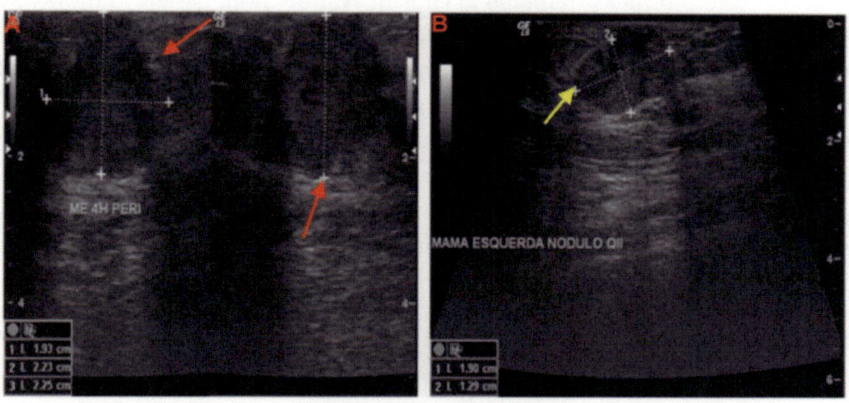

Figure 6. Breast ultrasound. A. Pretreatment: Node irregular, margin not circumscribed, hypoechoic, with posterior acoustic shadow in the left breast (red arrow). B. Post-treatment: Node with the same characteristics (yellow arrow), with inadequate response

5. Magnetic resonance imaging

Recently, magnetic resonance appeared in the list of imaging tests to be ordered, in the treatment of breast cancer. It has low specificity, because it presents difficulties in identification between benign and malignant lesions [33]. However, additional studies are needed to better characterize the resonance as an effective method in the determination of tumor extent. Magnetic resonance imaging has a sensitivity of 95-97% for the evaluation of lesions of less than 1 cm. It is important to detect disease in the contralateral breast (4% to 24% of associated disease). Magnetic resonance imaging increases the accuracy of radiology evaluated in monitoring response to chemotherapy, therefore it is relevant in the evaluation of a possible conservative surgery [34].

There is a significant disparity in mammography, breast ultrasound and MRI as compared methods in the evaluation of breast tumors. However, to relate them to the anatomopathological study, there is a greater difference between the measurements of ultrasound and mammography and a smaller difference between measurements made by MRI [35]. The accuracy of tumor measurement is fundamental in preoperative assessment when conservative treatment is desired. From a diagnostic point of view, physical examination, mammography, ultrasound and MRI have an accuracy in predicting pathologic response of 75, 89, 82 and 89% respectively [36]. Furthermore, studies comparing the various methods of images show a trend in favor of resonance, with better magnitude of correlation to anatomopathology exam [37].

According to a study of Matthes et al. [38] in 50 patients with locally advanced breast cancer before surgery, mammography and breast ultrasound showed no significant correlation. The MRI showed a moderate and significant correlation, suggesting to be a more reliable exam in relation to referred measurements in clinical examination. Others authors have shown good correlation between the anatomopathological and physical examination (0.68) while mammography and breast ultrasound were not good methods, with weak correlations ($r = 0.33$ and $r = 0.29$). However, Weatherall [39] suggests a high correlation for MRI ($r = 0.93$), moderate for clinical examination ($r = 0.72$) and moderate, but lower for mammography (0.62). Also noted, that few cases were evaluated with breast ultrasound, not justifying this analysis. According Drew et al a conventional assessment of response to neoadjuvant chemotherapy by clinical or mammographic methods presents many limitations for surgical planning [40].

In general, most studies showed that MRI allows a better assessment of tumors in relation to others tests, varying the index of correlation between $r = 0.60$ to 0.98 [37,41].

The studies demonstrate a tendency for MRI as an ideal method in the detection of carcinomas reaching the sensitivity of up to 100%. As was demonstrated by Matthes et al. [38], in most cases, MRI demonstrated a better correlation than the other imaging exams in the definition of tumor measurement after neoadjuvant chemotherapy. Yeh [42] conducted a comparison between diagnostic methods and concluded that MRI showed better correlation with pathology in relation to mammography and breast ultrasound. However, this showed that the exam could overestimate measurement of residual tumor in 6% of cases and underestimate them in up to 23%.

We must consider in the literature, that the MRI has a high correlation, but is not able to precisely identify the residual lesion in all cases, which justifies the preoperative marking of the area to be resected, especially in the LABC and when assessing the possibility of conservative treatment, resection of the entire enclosed area, seeing that, there is no data methodologically consistent in literature that ensures the assessment of residual lesion.

http://dx.doi.org/10.5772/53123

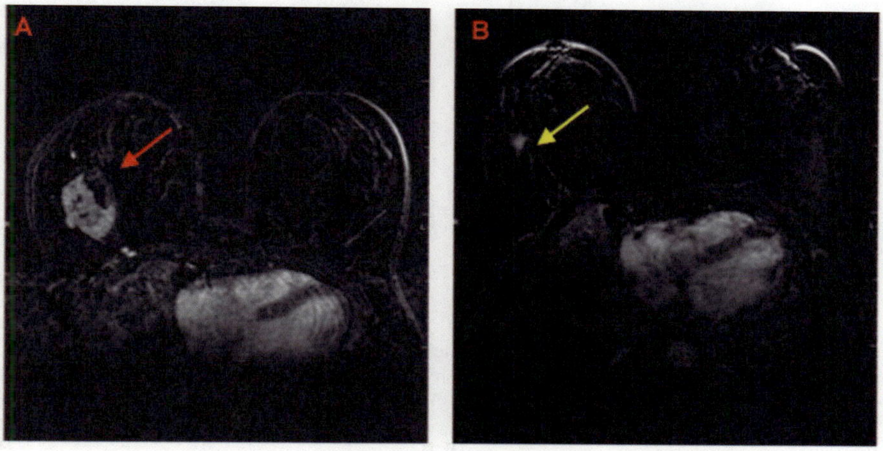

Figure 7. Breast MRI: A. Pretreatment: large tumor mass in the right breast (red arrow). B. Post-treatment: a nodular small area starting at the same topography (yellow arrow), showing a concentric reduction and partial tumor

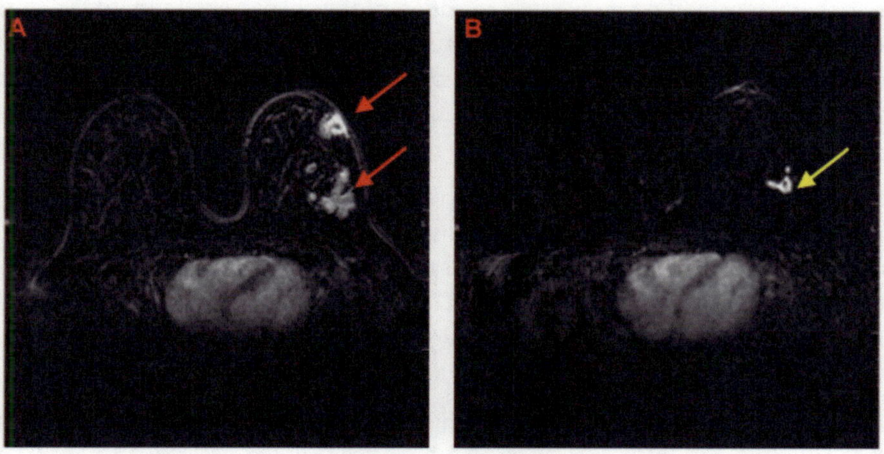

Figure 8. Breast MRI. A. Pretreatment: two masses in left breast (red arrow). B. Post-treatment: single mass in the left breast (yellow arrow), with partial tumor reduction.

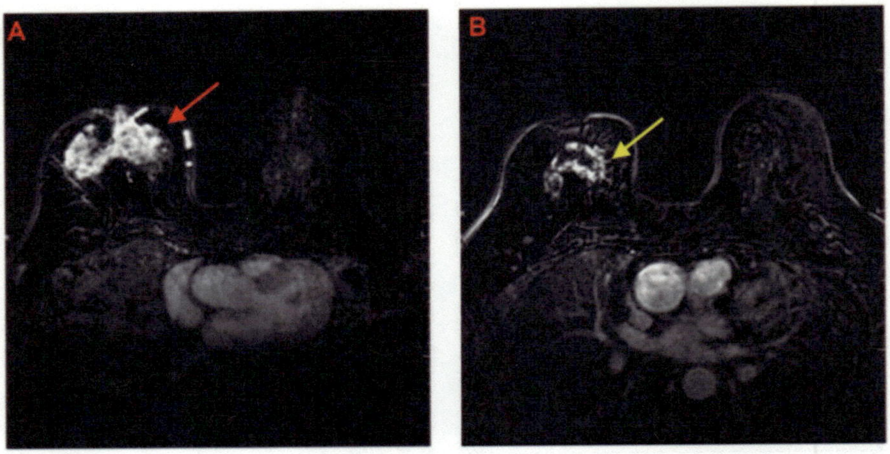

Figure 9. Breast MRI. A. Pretreatment: large mass in the right breast (red arrow). B. Post-treatment: mass in the right breast (yellow arrow), with partial reduction and diffuse tumor.

6. ^{99m}Tc- sestamibi scintigraphy

Nuclear medicine offers a noninvasive detection of histological, molecular and biochemical markers known to tumor aggressiveness and resistance to therapy, which can provide criteria for better therapeutic conduct [43].

Breast scintigraphy is a well-established diagnostic imaging technique [44], of relatively low cost compared with positron emission tomography and magnetic resonance imaging. It can also be used as a method for evaluating the response of breast carcinoma to chemotherapy treatment, thereby providing an *in vivo* indication of the chemosensitivity of the tumor [45]. Tiling et al. [46] showed that PET and breast scintigraphy with ^{99m}Tc-sestamibi are equivalent in monitoring the tumor response to neoadjuvant chemotherapy, with significant advantage of scintigraphy in the availability of the radiopharmaceutical and gamma cameras, besides a low cost.

The mechanism of ^{99m}Tc-sestamibi concentration in tumors is not entirely clear. It is distributed in the tissues in proportion to blood flow and enters cells by passive diffusion. By the transmembrane potential difference it is fixed to the mitochondria, particularly in malignant cells with higher negative potentials [47,48]. The highest accumulation in the lesion depends on mitochondrial activity and density, cellularity, angiogenesis and malformed vessels [49]. Factors of cell proliferation and desmoplastic activity seem to be involved [50].

The characteristics that lead to the accumulation of this radiopharmaceutical are identical to those that promote the inflow of chemotherapeutics, related directly to blood flow and transmembrane potential and negative mitochondrial and inversely with necrosis or fibrosis [47,51], and good correlation was observed between reduced uptake of ^{99m}Tc-sestamibi and the response to chemotherapy in LABC [52].

Mechanisms of accumulation and efflux of ^{99m}Tc-sestamibi in breast carcinomas involve cellular processes that are important in tumor response to treatment. Figure 10 shows the main relationships of accumulation and of the kinetics of ^{99m}Tc-sestamibi in the tumor and mechanisms of related chemoresistance.

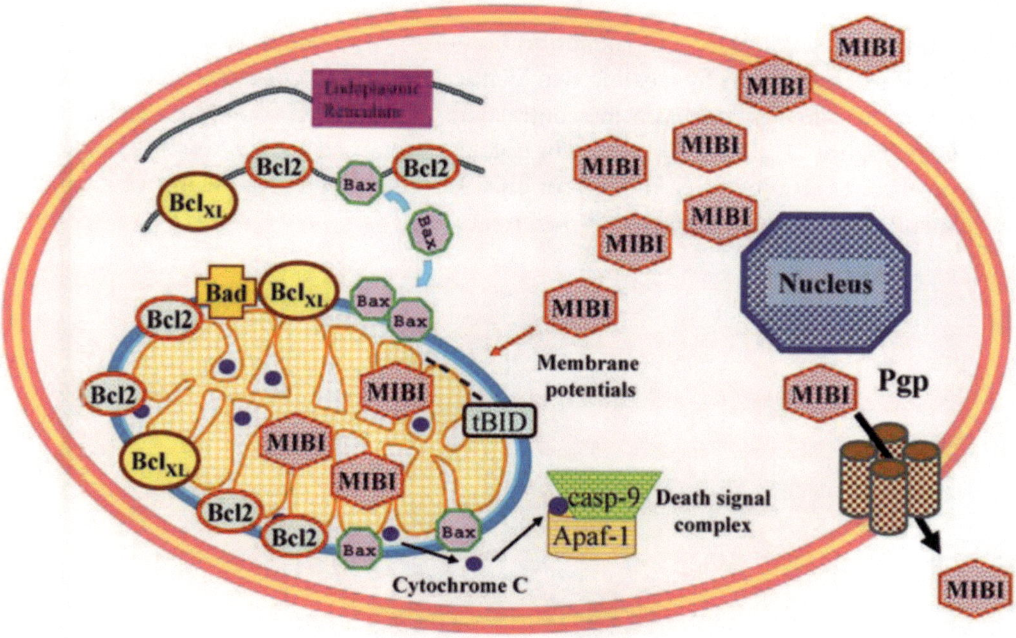

Figure 10. Schematic representation of uptake and efflux of ^{99m}Tc-sestamibi [43].

The mitochondrial membrane permeability is regulated by members of anti and pro-apoptotic of the Bcl-2 family [53]. When a signal of apoptosis converges to the mitochondrion, this causes an early increase in mitochondrial membrane permeability, release of cytochrome-c and other apoptotic factors [54] which trigger the activation of caspases, increasing the breaking of the cell substrate, causing morphological and biochemical changes characteristics of the apoptosis [55].

Due to the characteristics of mitochondrial accumulation of ^{99m}Tc-sestamibi, breast carcinomas that represent reduction of its inflow have high levels of anti-apoptotic protein Bcl-2 [56], which lead to resistance to chemotherapeutic agents and radiation due to the defect in the apoptosis [57]. Levels of Bcl-2 in breast carcinomas range from 32 to 86% [58]. Some studies report that the absence of Bcl-2 in LABCis associated with better chemotherapy response [59-61].

The efflux of ^{99m}Tc-sestamibi and wide variety of drugs of the cytoplasm to the extracellular matrix is related to P-glycoprotein. The over-expression of this protein is inversely related to the accumulation of ^{99m}Tc-sestamibi and with residual tumor in anatomopathological exams of surgical specimen, indicating inadequate response to neoadjuvant chemotherapy. Takamura et al [62], Alonso et al [63] and Sciuto et al [64] showed that breast scintigraphy with ^{99m}Tc-sestamibi, by analysis of washout of this in delayed images can be used as a predictor of neoadjuvant chemotherapy response. Early and increased concentration of ^{99m}Tc-sestamibi in breast carcinomas is associated with high proliferation rate, indicating more aggressive tumor behavior, and better and faster tumor response [43].

In the study of Koga et al [65], the quantification of ^{99m}Tc-sestamibi uptake is done on the lateral images of the breasts by creating two identical areas of interest: one on the tumor and the other in the mirror position on the contralateral breast. Pixel counting is performed in these areas (Figure 11). The ^{99m}Tc-sestamibi uptake rate caused by the tumor is determined as the pixel count ratio between the area of interest in the tumor and the mirror area in the contralateral breast in pretreatment and post-treatment.

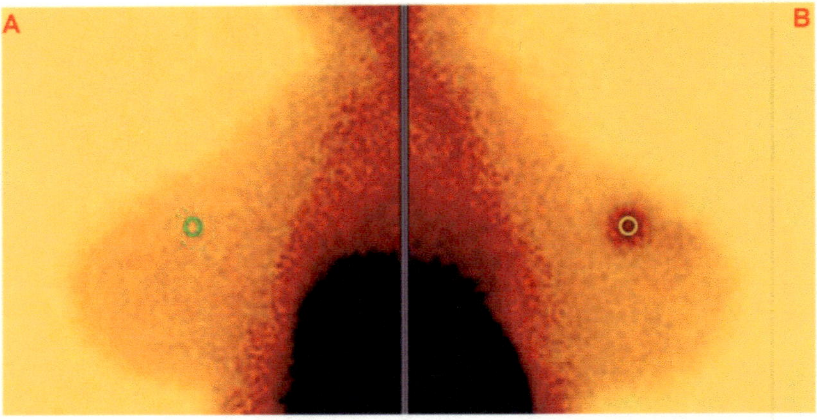

Figure 11. Breast scintigraphy. A. Left lateral: the mirror area in the contralateral breast (green circle). B. Right lateral: the area of interest in the tumor (yellow circle).

A better response to chemotherapy regimen was observed in more aggressive tumors that represent a higher uptake rate reduction. The tumor necrosis resulting from chemotherapy could explain the substantial reduction in tumor size [65]. The invasive ductal carcinoma presents a higher uptake rate reduction compared to those associated to the *in situ* component. Moriguchi et al [66] lower rates were found in ductal carcinomas *in situ* and mucinous probably related to lower cellular proliferation. This findings reflects the routine of oncological therapy, low response, carcinoma *in situ* to chemotherapy, confirming the utility of the rate in the evaluation of chemotherapy response in the different carcinoma groups.

Koga et al [65], Mankoff et al [67], Marshall et al [68] and Cwikla et al [69] reported a reduction of the rate of tumor:background, showing that the concentration of ^{99m}Tc-sestamibi reflects the metabolic activity of the tumor and its reduction resulting from chemotherapy [68]. Koga et al [65], Wilczek et al [70] showed a significant reduction rate of tumor: back-

http://dx.doi.org/10.5772/53123

ground after completion of neoadjuvant chemotherapy, confirmed by tumor regression in histological study of the surgical specimen.

Quantitative analysis on ^{99m}Tc-sestamibi scintigraphy is shown to be an additional tool for evaluating the preoperative chemotherapy response, given that the variation in ^{99m}Tc-sestamibi uptake reflects the biological behavior of the tumor [65].

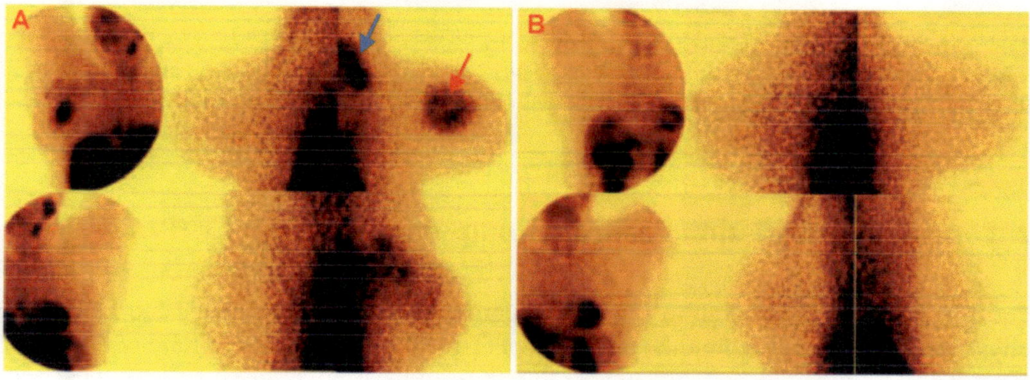

Figure 12 Breast scintigraphy. A. Pretreatment: large nodular area in right breast (red arrow) and ipsilateral axillary lymph node (blue arrow). B. Post-treatment: disappearance of the areas in breast and axillary lymph node, setting good response to neoadjuvant chemotherapy.

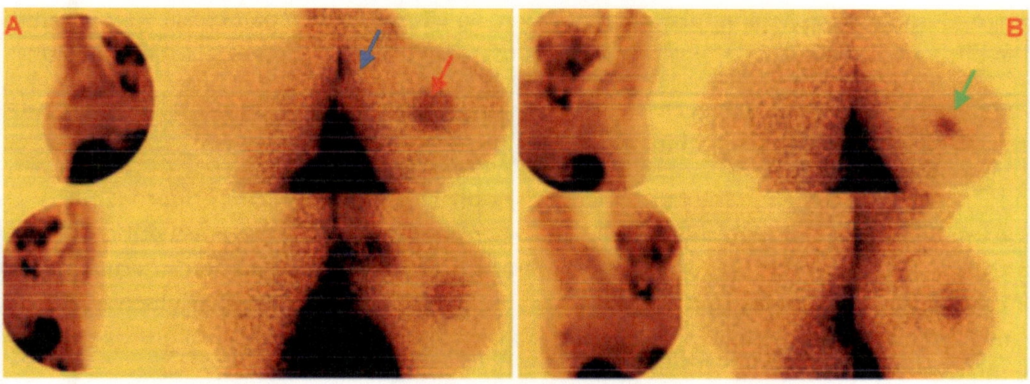

Figure 13 Breast scintigraphy. A. Pretreatment: large nodular area in right breast (red arrow) and ipsilateral axillary lymph node (blue arrow). B. Post-treatment: nodular area reduction in breast (green arrow) and axillary lymph node disappearance, setting partial response to neoadjuvant chemotherapy.

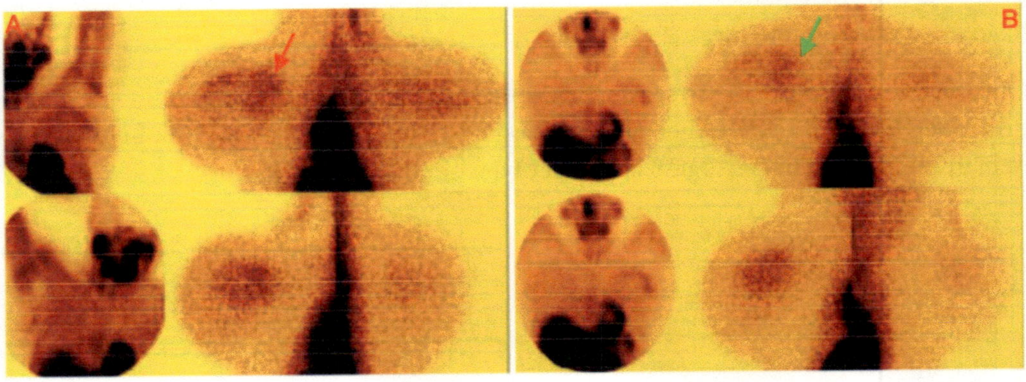

Figure 14. Breast scintigraphy. A. Pretreatment: large nodular area in left breast (red arrow). B. Post-treatment: nodular area unchanged (green arrow), configuring inadequate response to neoadjuvant chemotherapy.

7. Tomography Emission Positron/ Computed Tomography (PET/CT)

Positron Emission Tomography (PET) is a powerful technique to image biochemical or physiological processes within the body. The metabolic and biological activity of disease always precedes any anatomic evidence of the illness. PET is a biological imaging technique does not replace anatomical imaging as X Ray, computed tomography (CT) or magnetic resonance imaging (MRI), but adds the characterization of simple molecular process that are taking place in normal or diseased tissues within the body.

Positron is an antiparticle of the electron. When it is spelled from the nucleous of an atom, it travel only a short distance. During this travel across several millimeters, adjacent atoms are ionized and the positron loses energy and slow down. Positron then pairs up with an electron and undergoing an annihilation interaction, which produces a pair of 511 KeV annihilation photons that travel in opposite directions reaching PET radiation detectors for imaging.

The fusion of PET and CT images is very useful in the correlation of the exact site of anatomical and physiological information.

In PET oncologic imaging, the most widely radiopharmaceutical is 2-[^{18}F]-fluoro-2-deoxy-D-glucose (^{18}F-FDG). Biochemically ^{18}F-FDG is a nonphysiological compound with a chemical structure very similar to that of naturally occurring glucose; it serves as an external marker of cellular glucose metabolism. The ability no noninvasively image cellular glucose metabolism is important in oncological applications because many cancer cells use glucose at higher rates.

The absolute quantitative radiotracer uptake in tumor can be measured in an effort to differentiate between malignant and benign tissue. Named *Standard Uptake Value* (SUV) it can be useful in measuring tumor metabolic function [71].

Breast tumors have many phenotypical characters, as increase of vascularization and local permeability, increase of glycolitic metabolism and protein production, receptors expression, ADN proliferation index and hypoxia. All these factors can be evaluated by PET scan. The radiopharmaceutical more common for that purpose is ^{18}F-FDG.

^{18}F-FDG has been evaluated for diagnosis, staging (Figure 15) and restaging, monitoring therapy response and prognostication in patients with breast cancer [72].

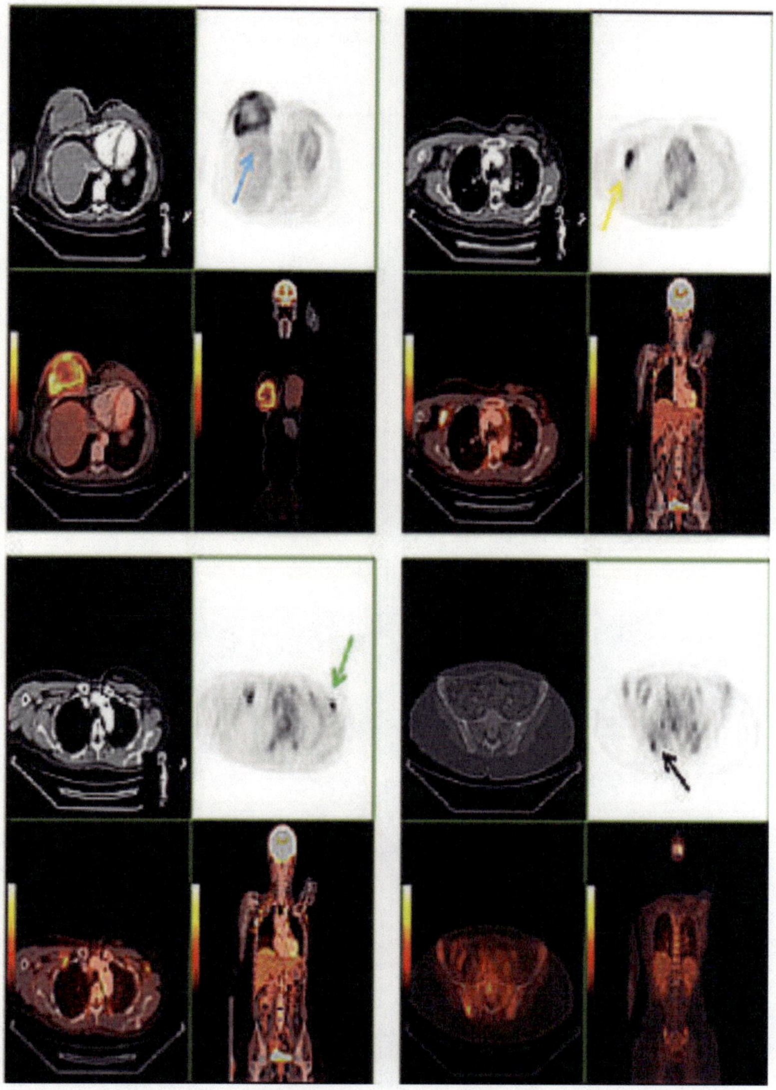

Figure 15. Staging of breast cancer. Female, 30 years old, follow up of right breast nodule for five years. Detected breast carcinoma by recent biopsy. PET/CT for staging identified metabolic hyperactivity in right breast carcinoma (blue arrow), many axillary (yellow arrow) and subpectoral lymph nodes (green arrow), mediastinum and bone lesions (black arrow).

Most studies evaluating ^{18}F-FDG to assess response to neoadjuvant therapy have measured change in ^{18}F-FDG uptake at mid-therapy, compared with at baseline, as a measure of response. Later, many studies found that ^{18}F-FDG uptake declines by aproximately 50% or more was predictive of a good response. Perhaps more important, lesser declines in ^{18}F-FDG uptake predicted poor response [73,74].

For analysis after the completion of chemotherapy, ^{18}F-FDG has shown that although residual ^{18}F-FDG uptake, predicts residual disease, but the absence of ^{18}F-FDG is not a reliable indicator of complete response, specially in lymph node envolvements. The presence of ^{18}F-FDG is highly predictive of relapse, as showed in Figures 16, 17 and 18 [72].

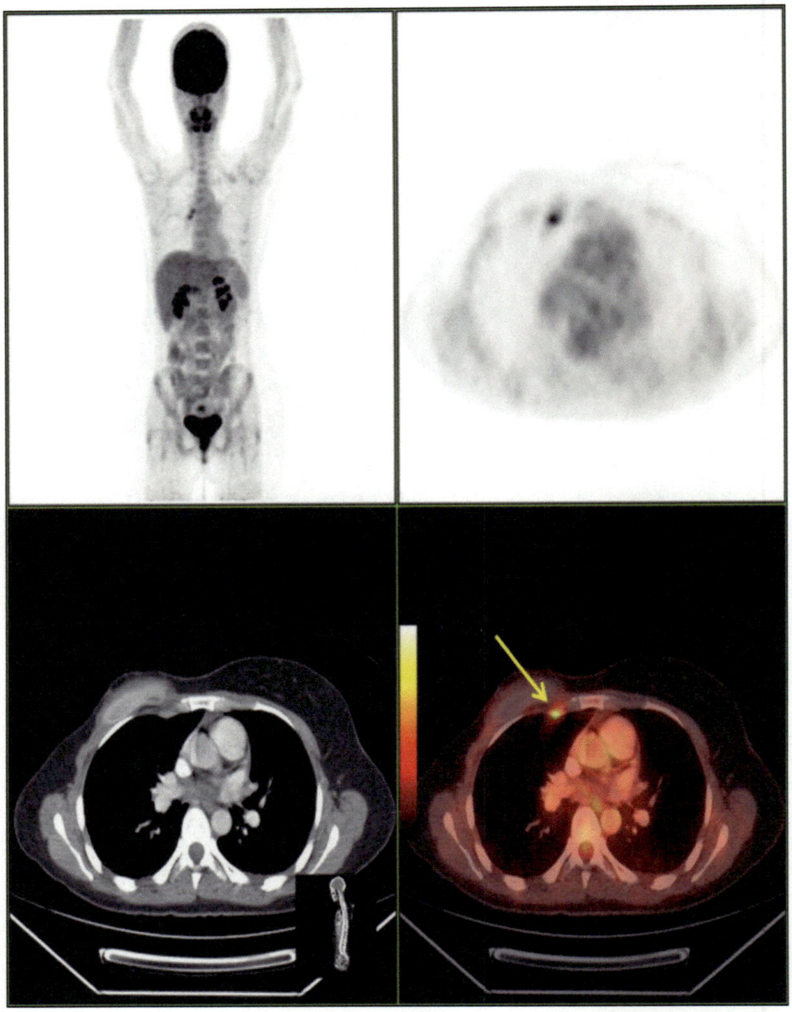

Figure 16. Recurrence of breast cancer. Female, 39 years old, with ductal carcinoma in right breast treated by radical mastectomy, chemotherapy and local radiotherapy two years ago. Follow up identified a nodulation in surgery bed. PET/CT showed metabolic activity in lymph node of internal mammary chair (yellow arrow).

http://dx.doi.org/10.5772/53123

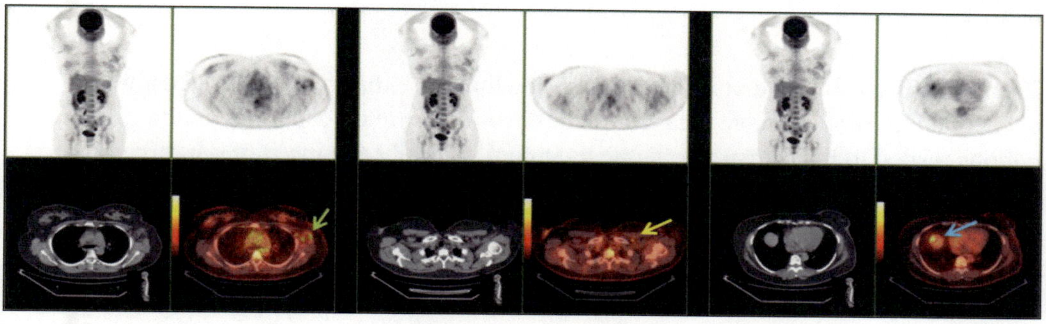

Figure 17. Disease progression. Female, 43 years old, with ductal carcinoma treated by left quadrantectomy and radiotherapy, chemotherapy and hormonetherapy two years ago. Follow up identified a nodule in left axillar region. PET/CT showed metabolic hyperactivity in axillary lymph nodes (green arrow), supraclavicular lymph nodes (yellow arrow) and in liver (blue arrow).

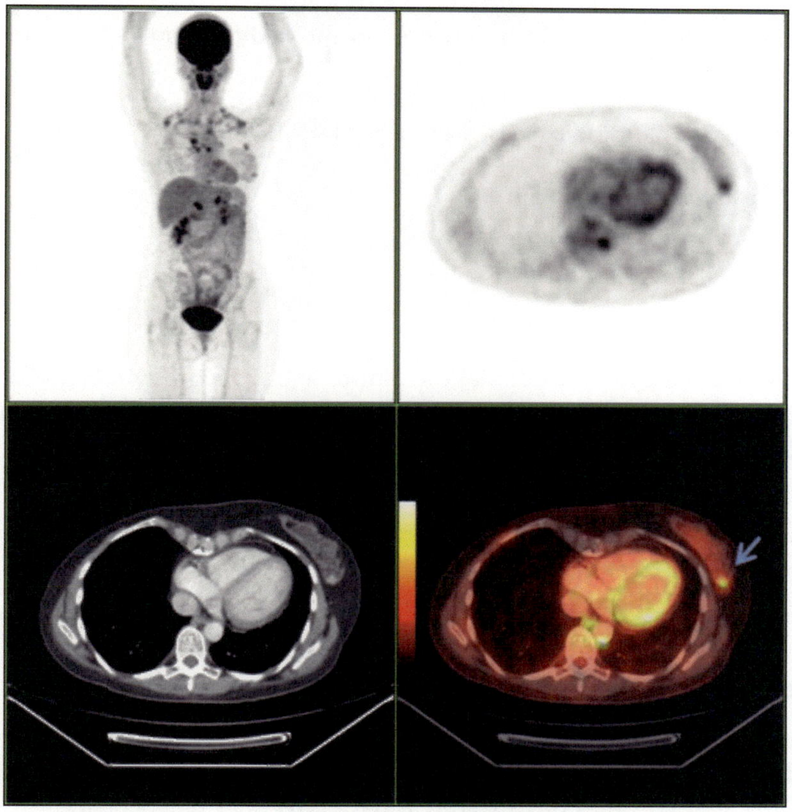

Figure 18. Follow up of breast cancer. Female, 46 years old, with ductal carcinoma in right breast treated by radical mastectomy, chemotherapy and local radiotherapy. Follow up Ca 19,9 levels increased. PET/CT showed metabolic activity in left breast identifying the second tumor (blue arrow).

8. Conclusions

There remains a shortage of information in the literature that confirms the best imaging exam for determining accurate measurements of residual tumor, especially in the case of evaluations related to the primary systemic treatment in locally advanced breast carcinoma.

Author details

Katia Hiromoto Koga[1*], Sonia Marta Moriguchi[1], Gilberto Uemura[2], José Ricardo Rodrigues[2], Eduardo Carvalho Pessoa[2], Angelo Gustavo Zucca Matthes[3] and Dilma Mariko Morita[4]

*Address all correspondence to: khkoga@.bol.com.br

1 Department of Tropical Diseases and Diagnostic Imaging, Botucatu Medical School – Sao Paulo State University, Brazil

2 Department of Gynecology and Obstretics, Botucatu Medical School – Sao Paulo State University, Brazil

3 Department of Mastology, Barretos Cancer Hospital, Brazil

4 DIMEN - Nuclear Medicine, Brazil

References

[1] INCA, Normas e Recomendações do Ministério da Saúde Controle do Câncer de Mama. Controle do câncer de mama - Documento de consenso. Rev Bras Cancerol. 2004; 50(2): 77-90.

[2] Elledge R M, Clark G M, Chamness GC, Osborne CK. Tumor biologic factors and breast cancer prognosis among white, Hispanic, and black women in the United States. J Natl Cancer Inst 1994; 86(9):705-12.

[3] Grabsch B., Clarke DM, Love A, et al. Psychological morbidity and quality of life in women with advanced breast cancer: a cross-sectional survey. Palliat Support Care 2006; 4(1):47-56.

[4] Lourenço TS, V. R., Mauad EC, Silva TB, Costa AM, Perez SV. Barreiras relacionadas a adesão ao exame de mamografia e rastreamento mamográfico da DRS-V do estado de São Paulo. Barreiras relacionadas a adesão ao exame de mamografia e rastreamento mamográfico da DRS-V do estado de São Paulo. Rev Bras Mastol 2009; 19(1):02-09.

[5] Jemal A, Siegel R, Ward E,et al. Cancer statistics, 2007. CA Cancer J Clin 2007; 57(1): 43-66.

[6] Sobin LH. UICC: TNM classification of malignant tumors. 2002

[7] Vieira RAC, M. A., Bailao Jr A, Fregnani CMS, Gonçalves BCJ, Borges AKN, Uemura G, Folgueira MAAK. Papel da tomografia computadorizada abdominal e torácica no estadiamento de tumores mamários localmente avançados. Rev Bras Mastol 2009; 19(1).

[8] Hortobagyi GN, Spanos W, Montague E, Buzdar AU, Yap HY, Blumenschein GR. Treatment of locoregionally advanced breast cancer with surgery, radiotherapy and combination chemoimmunotherapy. Int J Radiat Oncol Biol Phys 1983; 9:643-50.

[9] Hortobagyi GN. Multidisciplinary management of advanced primary and metastatic breast cancer. Cancer 1994; 74(1 suppl):416-23.

[10] Hortobagyi GN, Blumenschein GR, Spanos W, Montague ED, Buzdar AU, Yap HY, et al. Multimodal treatment of locoregionally advanced breast cancer. Cancer 1983; 51:763-8.

[11] Fisher B., Bryant J, Wolmark N.,et al. Effect of preoperative chemotherapy on the outcome of women with operable breast cancer. J Clin Oncol 1998; 16(8):2672-85.

[12] Mathew J, Asgeirsson K S, Cheung KL, et al. Neoadjuvant chemotherapy for locally advanced breast cancer: a review of the literature and future directions. Eur J Surg Oncol 2009; 35:113-22.

[13] Liu SV, Melstrom L, Yao K. Russell CA, Sener SF, et al. Neoadjuvant therapy for breast cancer. J Surg Oncol 2010; 101(4):283-91.

[14] Fuster D, Munoz M, Pavia J, Palacin A, Bellet N, Mateos JJ, et al. Quantified ^{99m}Tc-MIBI scintigraphy for predicting chemotherapy response in breast cancer patients: factors that influence the level of ^{99m}Tc-MIBI uptake. Nucl Med Commun 2002; 23:31-8.

[15] Lehnert M. Clinical multidrug resistance in cancer: a multifactorial problem. Eur J Cancer 1996; 6:912-20.

[16] Goldstein LJ. MDR1 gene expression in solid tumors. Eur J Cancer 1996; 32A:1039-50.

[17] Goldstein LJ, Galski H, Fojo A, Willingham M, Lai SL, Gazdar A, et al. Expression of a multidrug resistance gene in human cancer. J Natl Cancer Inst 1989; 81:116-24.

[18] Kieth WN, Stallard S, Brown R. Expression of MDR1 and GST-p in human breast tumors: comparison to in vitro chemosensitivity. Br J Cancer 1990; 61:712-6.

[19] Smith IC, Heys SD, Hutcheon AW, et al. Neoadjuvant chemotherapy in breast cancer: significantly enhanced response with docetaxel. J Clin Oncol 2002; 20(6):1456-66.

[20] Von Minckwitz G, Blohmer JU, Raab, et al. In vivo chemosensitivity-adapted preoperative chemotherapy in patients with early-stage breast cancer: the GEPARTRIO pilot study. Ann Oncol 2005; 16(1):56-63.

[21] Kaufmann M, Hortobagyi GN, Goldhirsch A, et al. Recommendations from an international expert panel on the use of neoadjuvant (primary) systemic treatment of operable breast cancer: an update. J Clin Oncol 2006; 24(12):1940-9.

[22] Prasad, SR, Saini S, Sumner JE, et al. Radiological measurement of breast cancer metastases to lung and liver: comparison between WHO (bidimensional) and RECIST (unidimensional) guidelines. J Comput Assist Tomogr 2003; 27(3):380-4.

[23] Feldman LD, Hortobaygi GN, Buzdar AU, Ames FC, Blumenschein GR. Pathological assessment of response to induction chemotherapy in breast cancer. Cancer Res 1986; 46:2578-81.

[24] Cocconi G, DiBlasio B, Albert G, Basagni G, Botti E, Peracchia G. Problems in evaluating response of primary breast cancer to systemic therapy. Breast Cancer Res Treat 1984; 4:309-13.

[25] Segel MC, Paulus DD, Hortobagyi GN. Advanced primary breast cancer: assessment at mammography of response to induction chemotherapy. Radiology 1988; 169:49-54.

[26] Moskovic EC, Mansi JL, King DM, Murch CR, Smith E. Mammography in the assessment of response to medical treatment of large primary breast tumor. Clin Radiol 1993; 47:339-44.

[27] Herrada J, Iyer RB, Atkinson EN, Sneige N, Buzdar AU, Hortobagyi GN. Relative value of physical examination mammography and breast sonography in evaluating the size of the primary tumor and regional lymph node metastasis in women receiving neoadjuvant chemotherapy for locally advanced breast carcinoma. Clin Cancer Res 1997; 3:1565-9.

[28] Yang WT, Lam WW, Cheung H, Suen M, King WW, Metreweli C. Sonography, magnetic resonance imaging and mammography assessments of preoperative size of breast cancer. J. Ultrasound Med 1997; 16:791-7.

[29] Gram, IT, Funkhouser E, Tabar L. The Tabar classification of mammographic parenchymal patterns. Eur J Radiol 1997; 24(2):131-6.

[30] Fornage, BD, Toubas O, Morel M. Clinical, mammographic, and sonographic determination of preoperative breast cancer size. Cancer 1987; 60(4):765-71.

[31] Kumar A, Singh S, Pradhan S, Shukla RC, Ansari MA, Singh TB, Shyam R, Gupta S. Doppler ultrasound scoring to predict chemotherapeutic response in advanced breast cancer. World J SurgOncol 2007; 28(5):99.

[32] Kuo WH, Chen CN, Hsieh FJ, Shyu MK, Chang LY, Lee PH, et al. Biol 2008; 34(6): 857-66.

[33] Flickinger FW, Allison JD, Sherry RM, Wright JC. Differentiation of benign from malignant breast masses by time-intensity evaluation of contrast enhanced MRI. Magn Reson Imaging 1993;11(5):617-20.

[34] Kaplan J.B. Posttherapeutic magnetic resonance imaging 2005; 227-237

[35] Balu-Maestro C, Chapellier C, Bleuse A, et al. Imaging in evaluation of response to neoadjuvant breast cancer treatment benefits of MRI. Breast Cancer Res Treat 2002; 72(2):145-52.

[36] Prati R, Minami C A, Gorn JA, et al. Accuracy of clinical evaluation of locally advanced breast cancer in patients receiving neoadjuvant chemotherapy. Cancer 2009; 115(6): 1194-202.

[37] Schott AF, Roubidoux MA, Helvie MA, et al. Clinical and radiologic assessments to predict breast cancer pathologic complete response to neoadjuvant chemotherapy. Breast Cancer Res Treat 2005; 92(3):231-8.

[38] Matthes AGZ. Clinical,radiologic and pathologic evaluation of locally advanced breast cancer in patients submitted to neoadjuvant chemotherapy. PhD Thesis - Botucatu Medical School 2010.

[39] Weatherall PT, Evans GF, Metzger GJ, Saborrian MH, Leitch AM. MRI vs. histologic measurement of breast cancer following chemotherapy: comparison with x-ray mammography and palpation. J Magn Reson Imaging 2001; 13:868-875.

[40] Drew P J, Kerin MJ, Mahapatra T, et al. Evaluation of response to neoadjuvant chemoradiotherapy for locally advanced breast cancer with dynamic contrast-enhanced MRI of the breast. Eur J Surg Oncol 2001; 27(7):617-20.

[41] Harms SE, Flamig DP. MR imaging of the breast. J Magn Reson Imaging 1993; 3(1): 277-83.

[42] Yeh E, Slanetz P, Kopans DB, et al. Prospective comparison of mammography, sonography, and MRI in patients undergoing neoadjuvant chemotherapy for palpable breast cancer. AJR Am J Roentgenol 2005; 184(3):868-77.

[43] Del Vecchio S, Zannetti A, Fonti R, Iomelli F, Salvatore M. ^{99m}Tc-MIBI in the evaluation of breast câncer biology. In: Bomdardieri E, Bonadonna G, Gianni L, Editors. Breast Cancer Nuclear Medicine in Diagnosis and therapeutic options. Germany: Springer Berlin Heidelberg New York; 2008.p.71-81.

[44] Khalkhali I, Diggles LE, Tailefer R, Vandestreek PR, Peller PJ, Abdel-Nabi HH. Procedure guideline for breast scintigraphy. J Nucl Med 1999; 40:1233-4.

[45] Hortobagyi GN. Comprehensive management of locally advanced breast cancer. Cancer 1990; 66:1387-91.

[46] Tiling R, Linke R, Untch M, Richter A, Fieber S, Brinkbäumer K, et al. 18F-FDG PET and 99mTc-sestamibi scintimammography for monitoring breast cancer response to neoadjuvant chemotherapy: a comparative study. Eur J Nucl Med 2001; 28:711-20.

[47] Fwnica-Worms D, Kronauge JF, Chiu ML. Uptake and retention of hexakis (2-methoxyisobutyl isonitrile) technetium(I) in cultured chick myocardial cells. Mitochondrial and plasma membrane potencial dependence. Circulation 1990; 82:1826-38.

[48] Chiu ML, Kronauge JF, Pwnica-Worms D. Effect of mitochondrial and plasma membrane potentials on accumulation of hexakis (2-methoxyisobutylisonitrile) technetium(I) in cultured mouse fibroblasts. J Nucl Med 1990; 31:1646-53.

[49] Omar WS, Eissa S, Moustafa H, Farag H, Ezzat I, Abdel-Dayam HM. Role of thallium-201 and Tc-99m-methoxy-isobutylisonitrile (Sestamibi) in evaluation of breast masses: correlations with immuhistochemical characteristic parameters (Ki-67, PCNA, Bcl-2 and angiogenesis) in malignant lesions. Anticancer Res 1997; 17:1639-44.

[50] Cutrone JA, Yospur LS, Khalkhali I, Tolmos J, Devito A, Diggles L, et al. Immunohistologic assessment of technetium-99m-MIBI uptake in benign and malignant breast lesions. J Nucl Med 1998; 39:449-53.

[51] Khalkhali I, Cutrone J, Mena I, Diggles L, Venegas R, Vargas H, et al. Technetium-99m-Sestamibi scintimammography of breast lesions: clinical and pathological follow-up. J. Nucl. Med 1995; 36:1784-9.

[52] Reyes R, Parbhoo SP, Cwikla JB, Buscombe JR, Jones AL, Hilson AJW. The role of scintimammography in prediction of response to primary chemotherapy. Eur J Cancer 2000; 36:S136.

[53] Cory S, Adams JM. The Bcl2 family: regulators of the cellular life-or-death switch. Nat Rev Cancer 2002; 2:647-56.

[54] Kroemer G, Reed JC. Mitochondrial control of cell death. Nat Med 2000; 6:513-9.

[55] Igney FH, Krammer PH. Death and anti-death: tumour resistance to apoptosis. Nat Rev Cancer 2002; 2:277-88.

[56] Del Vecchio S, Zannetti A, Aloj L, Caraco C, Ciarmiello A, Salvatore M. Inhibition of early ^{99m}Tc-MIBI uptake by Bcl-2 anti-apoptotic protein overexpression in untreated breast carcinoma. Eur J Nucl Med Mol Imaging 2003; 30:879-87.

[57] Reed JC. Drug Insight: cancer therapy strategies based on restoration of endogenous cell death mechanisms. Nat Clin Pract Oncol 2006; 3:388-98.

[58] Arun B, Kilic G, Yen C, Foster B, Yardley D, Gaynor R, et al. Correlation of bcl-2 and p53 expression in primary breast tumors and corresponding metastatic lymph nodes. Cancer 2003; 98:2554-9.

[59] Ogston KN, Miller ID, Schofield AC, Spyrantis A, Pavlidou E, Sarkar TK, et al. Can patients' likelihood of benefiting from primary chemotherapy for breast cancer be predicted before commencement of treatment? Breast Cancer Res Treat 2004; 86:181-9.

[60] Pusztai L, Krishnamurti S, Perez Cardona J, Sneige N, Esteva FJ, Volchenok M, et al. Expression of BAG-1 and BcL-2 proteins before and after neoadjuvant chemotherapy of locally advanced breast cancer. Cancer Invest 2004; 22:248-56.

[61] Prisack HB, Karreman C, Modlich O, Audretsch W, Danae M, Rezai M, et al. Predictive biological markers for response of invasive breast cancer to anthracycline/cyclophosphamide-based primary (radio-)chemotherapy. Anticancer Res 2005; 25:4615-21.

[62] Takamura Y, Miyoshi Y, Taguchi T, Noguchi S. Prediction of chemotherapeutic response by technetium 99m-MIBI scintigraphy in breast carcinoma patients. Cancer 2001; 92:232-9.

[63] Alonso O, Delgado L, Núñez M, Vargas C, Lopera J, Andruskevicius P, et al. Predictive value of ^{99m}Tc sestamibi scintigraphy in the evaluation of doxorubicin based chemotherapy response in patients with advanced breast cancer. Nucl Med Commum 2002; 23:765-71.

[64] Sciuto R, Pasqualoni R, Bergomi S, Petrilli G, Vici P, Belli F, et al. Prognostic value of 99mTc- sestamibi washout in predicting response of locally advanced breast cancer to neoadjuvant chemotherapy. J Nucl Med 2002; 43:745-51.

[65] Koga KH, Moriguchi SM, Neto JN, Peres SV, Silva ET, Sarri AJ, et al. ^{99m}Tc-sestamibi scintigraphy used to evaluate tumor response to neoadjuvant chemotherapy in locally advanced breast cancer: A quantitative analysis. Oncology Letters 2010; 1:379-82.

[66] Moriguchi SM, De Luca LA, Griva BL, Koga KH, Silva ET, Vespoli HL, et al. Accuracy of ^{99m}Tc-sestamibi scintimammography for breast cancer diagnosis. Experimental and Therapeutic Medicine 2010; 1:205-209.

[67] Mankoff DA, Dunnwald LK, Gralow JR, Ellis GK, Drucker MJ, Livingstone RB. Monitoring the response of patients with locally advanced breast carcinoma to neoadjuvant chemotherapy using [technetium 99m]- Sestamibi scintimammography. Cancer. 1999; 85:2410-23.

[68] Marshall C, Eremin J, Mohammed ES, Eremin O, Griffiths A. Monitoring the response of large (>3 cm) and locally advanced (T3-4, N0-2) breast cancer to neoadjuvant chemotherapy using ^{99m}Tc-Sestamibi uptake. Nucl Med Commun. 2005; 26(1): 9-15.

[69] Cwikla JB, Buscombe JR, Barlow RV, Kelleher SM, Parbhoo SP, Crow J, et al. The effect of chemotherapy on the uptake of technetium-99m Sestamibi in breast cancer. Eur J Nucl Med. 1997; 24:1175-8.

[70] Wilczek B, Von Schoultz E, Bergh J, Eriksson E, Larsson SA, Jacobsson H. Early assessment of neoadjuvant chemotherapy by FEC-courses of locally advanced breast cancer using ^{99m}Tc-MIBI. Acta Radiol. 2003; 43:284-7.

[71] Nuclear Medicine and PET/CT. Technology and Techniques. Seventh Edition. Edited by Paul E. Christian and Kristen M. Waterstram-Rich. Elsevier Mosby 2012, St Louis Missouri.

[72] Flanagan FL, Dehdashti F, Siegek BA. PET in breast cancer. Semin Nucl Med. 1998; 28: 290-302.

[73] Avril N, Sassen S and Roylance R. Response to therapy in breast cancer. J Nucl Med. 2009; 50: 55S-63S.

[74] Lee JH, Rose EL and Mankoff DA. Diagnosis and management of patients with breast cancer: Part 2 – Response to therapy, other indications, and future directions.. J Nucl Med, 2009, 50(5): 738-48.

Chapter 3

Neoadjuvant Chemotherapy for Breast Cancer

Suthiree Ithimakin and Suebwong Chuthapisith

Additional information is available at the end of the chapter

http://dx.doi.org/10.5772/53124

1. Introduction

1.1. Rationale of neoadjuvant chemotherapy in treatment of breast cancer

Neoadjuvant chemotherapy (NAC), also termed as preoperative, induction or primary chemotherapy, is defined as the administration of systemic chemotherapeutic agent prior to local control of surgery or radiation. Giving chemotherapy before performing a resection of tumour was initially introduced in locally advanced breast cancer where large inoperable tumour can be converted to operable cancer.

Moreover, at the time of breast cancer diagnosed with 2 to 3 cm in size, the risk of occult metastasis either in axillary lymph node or distant micrometastasis is greater than 50% [1], [2]. There were some evidences demonstrated in animal model that after surgical removal of primary cancer, metastases might be exacerbated [3], [4]. The administration of systemic chemotherapy in this setting might be a benefit to decrease the mortality risk from systemic spreading of the disease. Therefore, control of the disease prior to surgical treatment might produce a better treatment outcome. It was debated that NAC might delay the operation. However, the result from many studies showed that during the course of NAC breast cancer rarely progressed, or if it progressed that likely reflected the aggressive tumour which did not response to chemotherapy postoperatively.

Another main benefit of NAC is monitoring response to the treatment, so as a good model for *in vivo* test for the cytotoxic agents. The good response to NAC with complete pathological response (pCR) is a surrogate marker for overall survival. Recent advance in development of high potential but less toxicity chemotherapy as well as other targeted therapy has brought to higher rate of pCR. Significantly double increased rates of pCR was documented in breast cancer women who had docetaxel following 4 cycles of anthracycline-based NAC treatment, though overall survival (OS) was affected only if pCR in the breast and axillary nodes was achieved [5], [6]. The pCR rate was even higher in the addition of trastuzumab

INTECH
open science | open minds

and pertuzumab [7]. However, with recent breast cancer subtypes identifying by estrogen receptor (ER), progesterone receptor (PR) and HER-2 expression status documented in the recent St. Gallen guideline [8], pCR is likely associated with only in non-luminal subtype [9].

Furthermore, increased rate of breast conserving surgery (BCS) was documented in operable breast cancer with lower risk of local recurrence, in particular when pCR was achieved [10].

2. Neoadjuvant chemotherapy versus adjuvant chemotherapy

Preoperative or NAC has been compared with standard adjuvant chemotherapy as the treatment of breast cancer in several phase III studies. The primary end points mainly are disease-free survival (DFS) and OS. These studies showed that using the chemotherapy preoperatively did not improve DFS and OS, compared with using the same regimen as an adjuvant treatment. A pivotal study from the National Surgical Adjuvant Breast and Bowel Project (NSABP18) [11] compared the use of neoadjuvant adriamycin plus cyclophosphamide (AC) with the same regimen administering postoperatively. With 4-cycle of neoadjuvant AC, the complete clinical response rate (cCR) and pathological complete response rate (pCR) were 36% and 13%, respectively. In primarily operable breast cancer, NAC can downstage tumor and lead to small increase of breast conserving rate (60% vs 67%, p = 0.002). Although substantial response was found with neoadjuvant approach, there was no statistically significant difference in terms of DFS and OS at a 9-year follow up [12]. Another study from the European Organization for Research and Treatment of Cancer (EORTC) compared the efficacy of 5-fluorouracil, epirubicin and cyclophosphamide (FEC) preoperatively or postoperatively [13]. Consistent with the NSABP-B18 trial, the OS, PFS and relapse rate were similar between both groups. Also, several smaller studies exploring the benefit of NAC did not find any survival benefit for the neoadjuvant approach [13]-[15].

Recent meta-analysis addressed directly the benefit of neoadjuvant versus adjuvant chemotherapy [16]. This meta-analysis included nine randomized trials with the total of 3946 patients. There was no difference of death and disease progression. Surprisingly, the patients who received neoadjuvant treatment experienced higher local relapse (risk ratio of 1.22, p=0.015). This greater risk of local recurrence mainly occurred in the trials that the patients received radiotherapy without surgery in patients who achieved clinical complete response.

To date, the evidence-based literatures support the benefit of NAC as an approach to convert inoperable breast cancer to an operable tumor, or downstaging to increase breast conserving rate. These seems to be no difference in survival in patients with operable breast cancer whether chemotherapy is given before or after surgery.

3. Types of neoadjuvant chemotherapy for breast cancer

There was no inherent reason to believe that a regimen that works postoperatively will not work preoperatively. Therefore, a standard neoadjuvant regimen is an acceptable postoperative regimen. Previously, anthracycline-based chemotherapy was approved as standard of care for adjuvant treatment of operable breast cancer. It is justified to use at least three to four cycles of anthracycline-based regimen and additional cycles may be considered to maximize response. Later, combination of taxane and anthracycline using as an adjuvant treatment has been proven to be superior to anthracycline alone and become a standard of care in node-positive and high-risk node negative breast cancer. Therefore, several clinical trials have explored the different chemotherapy combinations using as the primary systemic treatment. The best type and schedule administration of preoperative taxanes were investigated in several phase III studies.

The study of NSABP-B27 is the largest study to demonstrate the benefit of adding docetaxel to anthracycine-based regimen [17]. Over 2000 patients were randomized to receive 1) 4 cycles of preoperative AC, 2) 4 cycles of neoadjuvant AC followed by 4 cycles of docetaxel and then surgery, and 3) 4 cycles of AC followed by surgery and then 4 cycles of adjuvant docetaxel. The results showed superiority of clinical response, pCR in patients who received the addition of docetaxel preoperatively (14% vs 26%, p<0.001), but similar breast conserving rate (63% vs 62%). Furthermore, adding docetaxel either preoperatively or postoperatively modestly reduced local recurrence rate with comparable DFS and OS [6].

In the Aberdeen trial, the locally-advanced breast cancer patients were initially treated with 4 cycles of the combination of cyclophosphamide, vincristine, adriamycin and prednisolone (CVAP). The patients who had response to CVAP were randomized to receive another 4 cycles of CVAP or 4 cycles of docetaxel. Among total 162 patients, 66 percent experienced clinical response following the CVAP. Of these, changing to docetaxel provided much better response rate (85% vs 64%, p=0.03), pCR rate (31% vs 15%, p=0.06) and 5-year survival rate (97% vs 78%, p=0.04) [18] .

Numerous trials have addressed to answer how best to incorporate taxane to anthracycline-based regimen. The German Preoperative Adriamycin and Docetaxel study II (GEPAR-DUO) [19] and the Arbeitsgemeinschaft Gastroenterologische Onkologie (AGO) study [20] explored whether using taxane sequentially or concurrently with anthracycline is the best approach. Both studies demonstrate significantly higher pCR and breast conserving rate in sequential arm. However, it is impossible to demonstrate that the better outcome of sequential arm is a result of sequential use itself or the higher cumulative dose of chemotherapy and longer duration of treatment with sequential administration. Another randomized study compared the efficacy of paclitaxel administered either weekly or every 3 weeks schedules, followed by the combination of 5-FU, adriamycin and cyclophosphamide (FAC). Weekly schedule associated with better pCR and also breast conserving rates [21].

Taken together, these data support the sequential use of anthracycline and taxane as the neoadjuvant treatment in both locally advanced and operable breast cancer. However, the usage of taxane in low-risk patients or ER-positive patients may provide minimal benefit outrage of the risk of adverse effect. Optimizing chemotherapy regimen should be considered individually based on reliable prognostic factor, patient's status and their preference after discussing of the risk and benefit of the treatment.

The patients who achieve poor response to initial neoadjuvant chemotherapy, i.e non-responder, have a worse prognosis. Modification of chemotherapy after observing poor response has not resulted in better outcome [22], [24]. In the German Preoperative Adriamycin and Docetaxel Study III (GEPAR-TRIO) study [22], the breast cancer patients who had poor response to 2 cycles of neoadjuvant docetaxel, adriamycin and cyclophosphamide (TAC) were randomized to receive another 4 cycles of TAC or alter to 4 cycles of vinorelbine plus capecitabine (NX). The results showed no difference in terms of breast conserving rate, clinical and pathological response. On the other hand, in the Aberdeen trial, the patients who received docetaxel after achieving poor respond to 4 cycles of cyclophosphamide, vincristine, doxorubicin and prednisolone (CVAP) ultimately had substantial overall response rate (66%) [25]. On the basis of limited benefit to neoadjuvant chemotherapy in non-responders, adjuvant therapy such as hormonal treatment as well as targeted therapy is considered as the standard treatment to improve outcome [26].

4. Other neoadjuvant therapies in treatment of breast cancer: evidence-based information

4.1. Neoadjuvant therapy for HER2-positive breast cancer

Overexpression of human epidermal growth factor receptor (HER2) is found in approximate 20-30 percent of breast cancer. Trastuzumab, a humanized antibody against HER2, combined with chemotherapy improved survival in metastatic HER2-positive breast cancer [27]. Moreover, 1-year of adjuvant trastuzumab has been established as standard treatment in HER2-positive breast cancer based on improvement of overall survival in several studies [28], [29]. With the promising activity of trastuzumab, its combination with neoadjuvant chemotherapy to enhance response has been proposed. There were several small phase II trials explored different combination of preoperative trastuzumab and chemotherapy. The pCR rate ranged from 12-45% [30], [31]. To date, there was a randomized controlled trial evaluated the efficacy of preoperative trastuzumab combined with anthracycline-based chemotherapy [32]. The stage II and III HER2-positive breast cancer patients were treated with 4 cycles of paclitaxel followed by 4 cycles of 5-fluorouracil, epirubicin and cyclophosphamide (FEC) with or without trastuzumab. The patients in trastuzumab arm had significantly higher pCR rate (65% vs 26%, p=0.016), but no difference in breast conserving rate. There was no incidence of clinical congestive heart failure. However, this study does not demonstrate whether preoperative trastuzumab impact survival compared to using trastuzumab postoperatively. Risk of cardiotoxicity and benefit of improving response are needed to be discussed individually.

Recently, there are several clinical trials comparing the efficacy of emerging anti-HER2, lapatinib and pertuzumab, as its efficacy using with chemotherapy or the addition to trastuzumab. The GeparQuinto trial compared the efficacy of lapatinib and trastuzumab, both concurrently with chemotherapy in operable HER2-positive breast cancer [33]. The pCR rate was significantly higher with the treatment of trastuzumab plus chemotherapy (30% vs 22%, p=0.04) However, breast conserving rate was not different and long-term outcomes are awaited. With the hypothesis of using dual anti-HER2 might inhibit HER2 receptor more efficiently, the clinical trials exploring the efficacy of dual anti-HER2, as neoadjuvant therapy in HER2-positive breast cancer were developed. Dual anti-HER2, eg. Lapatinib or pertuzumab plus trastuzumab, did increase pCR rate, but did not increase breast conserving rate compared to the patients who received trastuzumab plus chemotherapy. The studies of HER2-targeted therapy combined with chemotherapy as neoadjuvant setting in HER2-positive breast cancer are summarized in Table 1.

Studies	N	Treatment	pCR (%)	BCS (%)
Buzdar A et al*[32]	42	3wPx4->FECx4	26	53
		Same CMT+H	65	57
NOAH*[34]	235	CMT	20	NA
		CMT+H 1 year	39	
Neosphere*[7]	417	D+T	29	NA
		D+T+P	46	
		T+P	17	
		D+P	24	
Neoaltto*[35]	455	L->wP	25	31
		T->wP	30	28
		L+H->wP	51	26
GeparQuinto*[33]	620	ECx4->Dx4+H	30	63
		ECx4->Dx4+L	22	59

Abbrevations: N, number of patients; BCS, breast conserving rate; 3wP, Paclitaxel every 3 weeks; FEC, 5-FU+epirubicin +cyclophosphamide;H, Trastuzumab; CMT, chemotherapy; D, docetaxel; P, pertuzumab; L, lapatinib; wP, weekly paclitaxel; EC, epirubicin+cyclophosphamide; NA, not available; *The studies that reported significant different of pCR rate and breast conserving rate.

Table 1. Neoadjuvant therapy in HER2-positive breast cancer

4.2. Bevacizumab combined with chemotherapy as a neoadjuvant therapy in HER2-negative breast cancer

Bevacizumab, a monoclonal antibody against vascular endothelial growth factor, was shown to improve response rate and progression-free survival when added to chemotherapy in metastatic HER2-negative breast cancer patients [36], [37]. Two recent phase III trials [38], [39] determined whether the addition of bevacizumab to chemotherapy would increase pCR rate in HER2-negative operable breast cancer. Both studies confirmed that bevacizumab did increase pCR rate. However, there was a controversial result whether which specific subgroups would gain benefit from bevacizumab. It was claimed that bevacizumab added benefit in terms of pCR in only triple-negative patients from GeparQuinto trial [39], whereas only patients with positive estrogen receptor from the NSABP-B40 trial had higher pCR rate following bevacizumab treatment [38]. Because of contradictory results of these trials with premature long-term data as well as economic argument, therefore, bevacizumab is not recommended for neoadjuvant treatment in non-metastatic HER2-negative breast cancer.

4.3. Neoadjuvant endocrine therapy

Endocrine therapy has been used as a standard treatment in metastatic ER-positive breast cancer with the objective response of 30-40 percent. Because of low profile of toxicity, it is commonly used as the first option in low-risk metastatic breast cancer, ie asymptomatic, long disease-free interval and limited metastatic disease. Conversely, neoadjuvant endocrine therapy is not recommended as a standard of care because of its lower response rate compared with response rate in the study of neoadjuvant chemotherapy. The small studies reported response rate of 0-2 percent following tamoxifen [40], [41] and 2-3 percent after aromatase inhibitor treatment [40], [42]. The studies of neoadjuvant endocrine therapy are summarized in Table 2.

Studies	N	treatment	ORR (%)	BCS (%)
Eiermann et al*[43]	337	Letrozole	55	45
		Tamoxifen	36	35
Smith et al [44]	330	Anastrozole	37	46
		Tamoxifen	36	22
		Combine	39	26
Ellis et al*[40]	324	Letrozole	60	48
		Tamoxifen	41	36

Abbreviations; N, number of patients; ORR, overall response rate; BCS, breast conserving surgery rate; *The randomized studies with the significant difference of overall response rate and breast conserving rate.

Table 2. Randomized trials comparing different neoadjuvant endocrine therapy

Although the objective response of primary endocrine treatment is not promising, endocrine therapy remains a reasonable option in selected ER-positive breast cancer patients, for instance, the elderly patients who are not suitable for chemotherapy, or has organ function impairment, or desires to avoid adverse effect from chemotherapy. According to a randomized study comparing the efficacy of neoadjuvant chemotherapy and aromatase inhibitor in postmenopausal ER-positive breast cancer patients, clinical response and pCR were not significantly different [45] . However, possibility of breast conserving surgery following primary endocrine treatment is still infrequent.

With the rationale of the superiority of aromatase inhibitor to tamoxifen in metastatic setting of postmenopausal woman with breast cancer, the study of aromatase inhibitor in neoadjuvant setting compared to tamoxifen has been performed. Several studies showed higher overall response rate and also breast conserving rate with aromatase inhibitor [40], [43], [44] .

http://dx.doi.org/10.5772/53124

At present, there are no data available about neoadjuvant endocrine therapy in premenopausal woman.

5. Predicting of response to NAC

Although, recent chemotherapeutic regimen for NAC treatment in breast cancer containing anthracycline followed sequentially by a taxane can produces the good clinical response rates [46]. A cPR is still less than 30% [46], [47]. However, these chemotherapeutic agents are associated with significant morbidity. Therefore, the main benefit would be maximum if it were possible to identify patients who are most likely to benefit from NAC before or shortly after commencing the treatment. Recently, various biotechnologies, including both imaging and biomolecular platforms, have been investigated in order to find novel biomarkers or tests to predict responses to NAC. These technologies include molecular imaging, PET-CT, scintigraphy, genomics and proteomic platforms [48]. However, there is not any promising result demonstrated so far.

Amongst the above technologies, the most recent and feasible is the use of magnetic resonance imaging (MRI) as a early predictor of response to NAC. In a recent systematic review study, where dynamic contrast enhanced (DCE) MRI performed pre and after 1-2 cycles of NAC were compared, good sensitivity and specificity in predicting response to NAC was demonstrated, depending on various MRI parameters used for interpretation. Substantial reductions in tumour volumecould be accurate parameters in discriminating responders and non-responders after 1-2 cycles of NAC [49].

PET-CT using 18 F-FDG seemed to be a good technology in predicting response to NAC due to its combination of anatomical and functional characteristics of cancer cells. However, in a small study comparing ability of PET-CT, MRI and ultrasonography in predicting response to NAC, MRI was superior to PET-CT and ultrasonography [50].

6. Summary

With the rationale of NAC in term of controlling distant or micrometastasis, NAC should be a good approach in breast cancer for both early and locally advanced disease. However, in some early breast cancer, addition of chemotherapy might be an overtreatment with more harmful than useful. Evidence from various clinical studies confirmed the benefit of NAC by avoiding mastectomy in some responders. In the recent day, therefore, use of NAC is the treatment of choice for locally advanced or some early breast cancer. Combination of NAC and other targeted therapy such as trastuzumab have given even better outcome. Finally, further research is still required in order to predict response to NAC as early as possible so that patient who would not respond well to NAC could be identified early and would allow seeking for the other treatment.

Author details

Suthinee Ithimakin[1] and Suebwong Chuthapisith[2]

1 Department of Internal Medicine, Faculty of Medicine Siriraj Hospital, Mahidol University, Bangkok, Thailand

2 Department of Surgery, Faculty of Medicine Siriraj Hospital, Mahidol University, Bangkok, Thailand

References

[1] Carter CL, Allen C, Henson DE: Relation of tumour size, lymph node status, and survival in 24,740 breast cancer cases, Cancer 1989, 63:181-187

[2] Koscielny S, Tubiana M, Le MG, Valleron AJ, Mouriesse H, Contesso G, Sarrazin D: Breast cancer: relationship between the size of the primary tumour and the probability of metastatic dissemination, Br J Cancer 1984, 49:709-715

[3] Fisher B, Saffer E, Rudock C, Coyle J, Gunduz N: Effect of local or systemic treatment prior to primary tumour removal on the production and response to a serum growth-stimulating factor in mice, Cancer Res 1989, 49:2002-2004

[4] O'Reilly MS, Holmgren L, Shing Y, Chen C, Rosenthal RA, Moses M, Lane WS, Cao Y, Sage EH, Folkman J: Angiostatin: a novel angiogenesis inhibitor that mediates the suppression of metastases by a Lewis lung carcinoma, Cell 1994, 79:315-328

[5] Kuerer HM, Newman LA, Smith TL, Ames FC, Hunt KK, Dhingra K, Theriault RL, Singh G, Binkley SM, Sneige N, Buchholz TA, Ross MI, McNeese MD, Buzdar AU, Hortobagyi GN, Singletary SE: Clinical course of breast cancer patients with complete pathologic primary tumor and axillary lymph node response to doxorubicin=based neoadjuvant chemotherapy, J Clin Oncol 1999, 17:460-469

[6] Bear HD, Anderson S, Smith RE, Geyer CE, Jr., Mamounas EP, Fisher B, Brown AM, Robidoux A, Margolese R, Kahlenberg MS, Paik S, Soran A, Wickerham DL, Wolmark N: Sequential preoperative or postoperative docetaxel added to preoperative doxorubicin plus cyclophosphamide for operable breast cancer:National Surgical Adjuvant Breast and Bowel Project Protocol B-27, J Clin Oncol 2006, 24:2019-2027

[7] Gianni L, Pienkowski T, Im YH, Roman L, Tseng LM, Liu MC, Lluch A, Staroslawska E, de la Haba-Rodriguez J, Im SA, Pedrini JL, Poirier B, Morandi P, Semiglazov V, Srimuninnimit V, Bianchi G, Szado T, Ratnayake J, Ross G, Valagussa P: Efficacy and safety of neoadjuvant pertuzumab and trastuzumab in women with locally advanced, inflammatory, or early HER2-positive breast cancer (NeoSphere): a randomised multicentre, open-label, phase 2 trial, Lancet Oncol 2012, 13:25-32

[8] Goldhirsch A, Wood WC, Coates AS, Gelber RD, Thurlimann B, Senn HJ, Panel m: Strategies for subtypes--dealing with the diversity of breast cancer: highlights of the St. Gallen International Expert Consensus on the Primary Therapy of Early Breast Cancer 2011, Ann Oncol 22:1736-1747

[9] von Minckwitz G, Untch M, Blohmer JU, Costa SD, Eidtmann H, Fasching PA, Gerber B, Eiermann W, Hilfrich J, Huober J, Jackisch C, Kaufmann M, Konecny GE, Denkert C, Nekljudova V, Mehta K, Loibl S: Definition and impact of pathologic complete response on prognosis after neoadjuvant chemotherapy in various intrinsic breast cancer subtypes, J Clin Oncol 2012, 30:1796-1804

[10] Caudle AS, Hunt KK: The neoadjuvant approach in breast cancer treatment: it is not just about chemotherapy anymore, Current opinion in obstetrics & gynecology 2011, 23:31-36

[11] Fisher B, Bryant J, Wolmark N, Mamounas E, Brown A, Fisher ER, Wickerham DL, Begovic M, DeCillis A, Robidoux A, Margolese RG, Cruz AB, Jr., Hoehn JL, Lees AW, Dimitrov NV, Bear HD: Effect of preoperative chemotherapy on the outcome of women with operable breast cancer, J Clin Oncol 1998, 16:2672-2685

[12] Wolmark N, Wang J, Mamounas E, Bryant J, Fisher B: Preoperative chemotherapy in patients with operable breast cancer: nine-year results from National Surgical Adjuvant Breast and Bowel Project B-18, J Natl Cancer Inst Monogr 2001, 96-102

[13] van der Hage JA, van de Velde CJ, Julien JP, Tubiana-Hulin M, Vandervelden C, Duchateau L: Preoperative chemotherapy in primary operable breast cancer: results from the European Organization for Research and Treatment of Cancer trial 10902, J Clin Oncol 2001, 19:4224-4237

[14] Gianni L, Baselga J, Eiermann W, Guillem Porta V, Semiglazov V, Lluch A, Zambetti M, Sabadell D, Raab G, Llombart Cussac A, Bozhok A, Martinez-Agullo A, Greco M, Byakhov M, Lopez Lopez JJ, Mansutti M, Valagussa P, Bonadonna G: Feasibility and tolerability of sequential doxorubicin/paclitaxel followed by cyclophosphamide, methotrexate, and fluorouracil and its effects on tumor response as preoperative therapy, Clin Cancer Res 2005, 11:8715-8721

[15] Scholl SM, Fourquet A, Asselain B, Pierga JY, Vilcoq JR, Durand JC, Dorval T, Palangie T, Jouve M, Beuzeboc P, et al.: Neoadjuvant versus adjuvant chemotherapy in premenopausal patients with tumours considered too large for breast conserving surgery: preliminary results of a randomised trial: S6, Eur J Cancer 1994, 30A:645-652

[16] Mauri D, Pavlidis N, Ioannidis JP: Neoadjuvant versus adjuvant systemic treatment in breast cancer: a meta-analysis, J Natl Cancer Inst 2005, 97:188-194

[17] Bear HD, Anderson S, Brown A, Smith R, Mamounas EP, Fisher B, Margolese R, Theoret H, Soran A, Wickerham DL, Wolmark N: The effect on tumor response of adding sequential preoperative docetaxel to preoperative doxorubicin and cyclophosphamide: preliminary results from National Surgical Adjuvant Breast and Bowel Project Protocol B-27, J Clin Oncol 2003, 21:4165-4174

[18] Heys SD, Hutcheon AW, Sarkar TK, Ogston KN, Miller ID, Payne S, Smith I, Walker LG, Eremin O: Neoadjuvant docetaxel in breast cancer: 3-year survival results from the Aberdeen trial, Clin Breast Cancer 2002, 3 Suppl 2:S69-74

[19] von Minckwitz G, Raab G, Caputo A, Schutte M, Hilfrich J, Blohmer JU, Gerber B, Costa SD, Merkle E, Eidtmann H, Lampe D, Jackisch C, du Bois A, Kaufmann M: Doxorubicin with cyclophosphamide followed by docetaxel every 21 days compared with doxorubicin and docetaxel every 14 days as preoperative treatment in operable breast cancer: the GEPARDUO study of the German Breast Group, J Clin Oncol 2005, 23:2676-2685

[20] Untch M, Mobus V, Kuhn W, Muck BR, Thomssen C, Bauerfeind I, Harbeck N, Werner C, Lebeau A, Schneeweiss A, Kahlert S, von Koch F, Petry KU, Wallwiener D, Kreienberg R, Albert US, Luck HJ, Hinke A, Janicke F, Konecny GE: Intensive dose-dense compared with conventionally scheduled preoperative chemotherapy for high-risk primary breast cancer, J Clin Oncol 2009, 27:2938-2945

[21] Green MC, Buzdar AU, Smith T, Ibrahim NK, Valero V, Rosales MF, Cristofanilli M, Booser DJ, Pusztai L, Rivera E, Theriault RL, Carter C, Frye D, Hunt KK, Symmans WF, Strom EA, Sahin AA, Sikov W, Hortobagyi GN: Weekly paclitaxel improves pathologic complete remission in operable breast cancer when compared with paclitaxel once every 3 weeks, J Clin Oncol 2005, 23:5983-5992

[22] von Minckwitz G, Kummel S, Vogel P, Hanusch C, Eidtmann H, Hilfrich J, Gerber B, Huober J, Costa SD, Jackisch C, Loibl S, Mehta K, Kaufmann M: Neoadjuvant vinorelbine-capecitabine versus docetaxel-doxorubicin-cyclophosphamide in early nonresponsive breast cancer: phase III randomized GeparTrio trial, J Natl Cancer Inst 2008, 100:542-551

[23] Thomas E, Holmes FA, Smith TL, Buzdar AU, Frye DK, Fraschini G, Singletary SE, Theriault RL, McNeese MD, Ames F, Walters R, Hortobagyi GN: The use of alternate, non-cross-resistant adjuvant chemotherapy on the basis of pathologic response to a neoadjuvant doxorubicin-based regimen in women with operable breast cancer: long-term results from a prospective randomized trial, J Clin Oncol 2004, 22:2294-2302

[24] Wesolowski R, Budd GT: Neoadjuvant therapy for breast cancer: assessing treatment progress and managing poor responders, Curr Oncol Rep 2009, 11:37-44

[25] Smith IC, Heys SD, Hutcheon AW, Miller ID, Payne S, Gilbert FJ, Ah-See AK, Eremin O, Walker LG, Sarkar TK, Eggleton SP, Ogston KN: Neoadjuvant chemotherapy in breast cancer: significantly enhanced response with docetaxel, J Clin Oncol 2002, 20:1456-1466

[26] Gralow JR, Burstein HJ, Wood W, Hortobagyi GN, Gianni L, von Minckwitz G, Buzdar AU, Smith IE, Symmans WF, Singh B, Winer EP: Preoperative therapy in invasive breast cancer: pathologic assessment and systemic therapy issues in operable disease, J Clin Oncol 2008, 26:814-819

[27] Slamon DJ, Leyland-Jones B, Shak S, Fuchs H, Paton V, Bajamonde A, Fleming T, Eiermann W, Wolter J, Pegram M, Baselga J, Norton L: Use of chemotherapy plus a monoclonal antibody against HER2 for metastatic breast cancer that overexpresses HER2, N Engl J Med 2001, 344:783-792

[28] Piccart-Gebhart MJ, Procter M, Leyland-Jones B, Goldhirsch A, Untch M, Smith I, Gianni L, Baselga J, Bell R, Jackisch C, Cameron D, Dowsett M, Barrios CH, Steger G, Huang CS, Andersson M, Inbar M, Lichinitser M, Lang I, Nitz U, Iwata H, Thomssen C, Lohrisch C, Suter TM, Ruschoff J, Suto T, Greatorex V, Ward C, Straehle C, McFadden E, Dolci MS, Gelber RD: Trastuzumab after adjuvant chemotherapy in HER2-positive breast cancer, N Engl J Med 2005, 353:1659-1672

[29] Romond EH, Perez EA, Bryant J, Suman VJ, Geyer CE, Jr., Davidson NE, Tan-Chiu E, Martino S, Paik S, Kaufman PA, Swain SM, Pisansky TM, Fehrenbacher L, Kutteh LA, Vogel VG, Visscher DW, Yothers G, Jenkins RB, Brown AM, Dakhil SR, Mamounas EP, Lingle WL, Klein PM, Ingle JN, Wolmark N: Trastuzumab plus adjuvant chemotherapy for operable HER2-positive breast cancer, N Engl J Med 2005, 353:1673-1684

[30] Burstein HJ, Harris LN, Gelman R, Lester SC, Nunes RA, Kaelin CM, Parker LM, Ellisen LW, Kuter I, Gadd MA, Christian RL, Kennedy PR, Borges VF, Bunnell CA, Younger J, Smith BL, Winer EP: Preoperative therapy with trastuzumab and paclitaxel followed by sequential adjuvant doxorubicin/cyclophosphamide for HER2 overexpressing stage II or III breast cancer: a pilot study, J Clin Oncol 2003, 21:46-53

[31] Wenzel C, Hussian D, Bartsch R, Pluschnig U, Locker GJ, Rudas M, Gnant MF, Jakesz R, Zielinkski CC, Steger GG: Preoperative therapy with epidoxorubicin and docetaxel plus trastuzumab in patients with primary breast cancer: a pilot study, J Cancer Res Clin Oncol 2004, 130:400-404

[32] Buzdar AU, Ibrahim NK, Francis D, Booser DJ, Thomas ES, Theriault RL, Pusztai L, Green MC, Arun BK, Giordano SH, Cristofanilli M, Frye DK, Smith TL, Hunt KK, Singletary SE, Sahin AA, Ewer MS, Buchholz TA, Berry D, Hortobagyi GN: Significantly higher pathologic complete remission rate after neoadjuvant therapy with trastuzumab, paclitaxel, and epirubicin chemotherapy: results of a randomized trial in human epidermal growth factor receptor 2-positive operable breast cancer, J Clin Oncol 2005, 23:3676-3685

[33] Untch M, Loibl S, Bischoff J, Eidtmann H, Kaufmann M, Blohmer JU, Hilfrich J, Strumberg D, Fasching PA, Kreienberg R, Tesch H, Hanusch C, Gerber B, Rezai M, Jackisch C, Huober J, Kuhn T, Nekljudova V, von Minckwitz G: Lapatinib versus trastuzumab in combination with neoadjuvant anthracycline-taxane-based chemotherapy (GeparQuinto, GBG 44): a randomised phase 3 trial, Lancet Oncol 2012, 13:135-144

[34] Gianni L, Eiermann W, Semiglazov V, Manikhas A, Lluch A, Tjulandin S, Zambetti M, Vazquez F, Byakhow M, Lichinitser M, Climent MA, Ciruelos E, Ojeda B, Mansut-

ti M, Bozhok A, Baronio R, Feyereislova A, Barton C, Valagussa P, Baselga J: Neoadjuvant chemotherapy with trastuzumab followed by adjuvant trastuzumab versus neoadjuvant chemotherapy alone, in patients with HER2-positive locally advanced breast cancer (the NOAH trial): a randomised controlled superiority trial with a parallel HER2-negative cohort, Lancet 2010, 375:377-384

[35] Baselga J, Bradbury I, Eidtmann H, Di Cosimo S, de Azambuja E, Aura C, Gomez H, Dinh P, Fauria K, Van Dooren V, Aktan G, Goldhirsch A, Chang TW, Horvath Z, Coccia-Portugal M, Domont J, Tseng LM, Kunz G, Sohn JH, Semiglazov V, Lerzo G, Palacova M, Probachai V, Pusztai L, Untch M, Gelber RD, Piccart-Gebhart M: Lapatinib with trastuzumab for HER2-positive early breast cancer (NeoALTTO): a randomised, open-label, multicentre, phase 3 trial, Lancet 2012, 379:633-640

[36] Miles DW, Chan A, Dirix LY, Cortes J, Pivot X, Tomczak P, Delozier T, Sohn JH, Provencher L, Puglisi F, Harbeck N, Steger GG, Schneeweiss A, Wardley AM, Chlistalla A, Romieu G: Phase III study of bevacizumab plus docetaxel compared with placebo plus docetaxel for the first-line treatment of human epidermal growth factor receptor 2-negative metastatic breast cancer, J Clin Oncol 2010, 28:3239-3247

[37] Miller K, Wang M, Gralow J, Dickler M, Cobleigh M, Perez EA, Shenkier T, Cella D, Davidson NE: Paclitaxel plus bevacizumab versus paclitaxel alone for metastatic breast cancer, N Engl J Med 2007, 357:2666-2676

[38] Bear HD, Tang G, Rastogi P, Geyer CE, Jr., Robidoux A, Atkins JN, Baez-Diaz L, Brufsky AM, Mehta RS, Fehrenbacher L, Young JA, Senecal FM, Gaur R, Margolese RG, Adams PT, Gross HM, Costantino JP, Swain SM, Mamounas EP, Wolmark N: Bevacizumab added to neoadjuvant chemotherapy for breast cancer, N Engl J Med 2012, 366:310-320

[39] von Minckwitz G, Eidtmann H, Rezai M, Fasching PA, Tesch H, Eggemann H, Schrader I, Kittel K, Hanusch C, Kreienberg R, Solbach C, Gerber B, Jackisch C, Kunz G, Blohmer JU, Huober J, Hauschild M, Fehm T, Muller BM, Denkert C, Loibl S, Nekljudova V, Untch M: Neoadjuvant chemotherapy and bevacizumab for HER2-negative breast cancer, N Engl J Med 2012, 366:299-309

[40] Ellis MJ, Coop A, Singh B, Mauriac L, Llombert-Cussac A, Janicke F, Miller WR, Evans DB, Dugan M, Brady C, Quebe-Fehling E, Borgs M: Letrozole is more effective neoadjuvant endocrine therapy than tamoxifen for ErbB-1- and/or ErbB-2-positive, estrogen receptor-positive primary breast cancer: evidence from a phase III randomized trial, J Clin Oncol 2001, 19:3808-3816

[41] Mauriac L, Debled M, Durand M, Floquet A, Boulanger V, Dagada C, Trufflandier N, MacGrogan G: Neoadjuvant tamoxifen for hormone-sensitive non-metastatic breast carcinomas in early postmenopausal women, Ann Oncol 2002, 13:293-298

[42] Barnadas A, Gil M, Gonzalez S, Tusquets I, Munoz M, Arcusa A, Prieto L, Margeli-Vila M, Moreno A: Exemestane as primary treatment of oestrogen receptor-positive

breast cancer in postmenopausal women: a phase II trial, Br J Cancer 2009, 100:442-449

[43] Eiermann W, Paepke S, Appfelstaedt J, Llombart-Cussac A, Eremin J, Vinholes J, Mauriac L, Ellis M, Lassus M, Chaudri-Ross HA, Dugan M, Borgs M: Preoperative treatment of postmenopausal breast cancer patients with letrozole: A randomized double-blind multicenter study, Ann Oncol 2001, 12:1527-1532

[44] Smith IE, Dowsett M, Ebbs SR, Dixon JM, Skene A, Blohmer JU, Ashley SE, Francis S, Boeddinghaus I, Walsh G: Neoadjuvant treatment of postmenopausal breast cancer with anastrozole, tamoxifen, or both in combination: the Immediate Preoperative Anastrozole, Tamoxifen, or Combined with Tamoxifen (IMPACT) multicenter double-blind randomized trial, J Clin Oncol 2005, 23:5108-5116

[45] Semiglazov VF, Semiglazov VV, Dashyan GA, Ziltsova EK, Ivanov VG, Bozhok AA, Melnikova OA, Paltuev RM, Kletzel A, Berstein LM: Phase 2 randomized trial of primary endocrine therapy versus chemotherapy in postmenopausal patients with estrogen receptor-positive breast cancer, Cancer 2007, 110:244-254

[46] Jones RL, Smith IE: Neoadjuvant treatment for early-stage breast cancer: opportunities to assess tumour response, Lancet Oncol 2006, 7:869-874

[47] Chollet P, Amat S, Cure H, de Latour M, Le Bouedec G, Mouret-Reynier MA, Ferriere JP, Achard JL, Dauplat J, Penault-Llorca F: Prognostic significance of a complete pathological response after induction chemotherapy in operable breast cancer, Br J Cancer 2002, 86:1041-1046

[48] Chuthapisith S, Eremin JM, Eremin O: Predicting response to neoadjuvant chemotherapy in breast cancer: molecular imaging, systemic biomarkers and the cancer metabolome (Review), Oncol Rep 2008, 20:699-703

[49] Marinovich ML, Sardanelli F, Ciatto S, Mamounas E, Brennan M, Macaskill P, Irwig L, von Minckwitz G, Houssami N: Early prediction of pathologic response to neoadjuvant therapy in breast cancer: Systematic review of the accuracy of MRI, Breast 2012,

[50] Choi JH, Lim HI, Lee SK, Kim WW, Kim SM, Cho E, Ko EY, Han BK, Park YH, Ahn JS, Im YH, Lee JE, Yang JH, Nam SJ: The role of PET CT to evaluate the response to neoadjuvant chemotherapy in advanced breast cancer: comparison with ultrasonography and magnetic resonance imaging, Journal of surgical oncology 2010, 102:392-397

Chapter 4

Neoadjuvant Chemotherapy: Role in Breast Cancer

Jasmeet Chadha Singh and Amy Tiersten

Additional information is available at the end of the chapter

http://dx.doi.org/10.5772/53192

1. Introduction

Neoadjuvant chemotherapy (NAC), also referred to as preoperative or primary chemotherapy refers to chemotherapy administered prior to tumor resection. It is a standard of care for management of locally advanced or inoperable breast tumors.

2. Rationale for NAC

The clinical rationale of NAC administration lies in the fact that it significantly downstages the existing tumor, enabling greater breast conservation (BSC). Although preoperative chemotherapy has not been shown to improve disease free (DFS) and overall survival (OS) for breast cancer when compared to post-operative therapy in operable patients, achievement of pathological complete response (pCR) defined as absence of any residual invasive tumor, is an important predictor of superior DFS and OS. In the B-27 trial looking at addition of taxanes to anthracycline based regimen in NAC, after 8 years of follow, patients who achieved pCR had superior DFS (HR: 0.49, $p<0.0001$) and OS (HR: 0.36, $P<0.0001$) rates. [1]- [5] The more recent I-SPY 1 study amongst several other studies [6]- [8], have found pCR to be an important predictor of recurrence free survival. [9], [10]

NSABP B-18 study was one of the earliest trials comparing neoadjuvant to adjuvant chemotherapy. The regimen of choice in this trial was the combination of adriamycin and cyclophosphamide (AC) either pre- or post operatively in 1523 women with operable palpable (T1-3, N0-1, M0) newly diagnosed breast cancer. There was no difference in overall survival between the two groups. However, a significantly greater number of patients underwent BCS in the NAC group (67vs. 60%, $p=0.002$).

In another trial of 1355 women with operable breast cancer, doxorubicin and paclitaxel followed by CMF in the neoadjuvant setting yielded similar RFS and OS rates when compared to adjuvant chemotherapy. However, patients with neoadjuvant chemotherapy achieved much higher breast conservation rates (63% vs. 34%, p<0.001). Distant relapse free survival was inferior in patients who did not achieve pCR (HR, 0.43; p- 0.025). [11]

3. Prognostic factors

Clinical trials have described various clinical and histological features of breast tumors, which may predict response to neoadjuvant chemotherapy. Higher nuclear grade is a significant predictor of pCR with NAC in several studies. [12]- [17] Proliferation index or Ki-67 [18] is shown to correlate positively to response. In the I SPY 1 trial, pCR rates in patients with high Ki-67 (defined as >20 percent) were 35% vs. 5% in patients with low Ki-67 (defined as <10 percent). [19] [9], [20] Pathologic examination of 82 breast cancer tumors after NAC with paclitaxel followed by 5-fluorouracil, adriyamicin and cyclophosphamide (T ▪ FAC) showed that basal like tumor pathology was a predictor of good response to NAC. [21] In the I SPY 1 trial luminal A histology had lowest pCR rates. [8], [19], [22] Negative estrogen and progesterone receptor status has shown to predict better response to NAC [7], [8], [13], [18], [23] In the I-SPY 1 trial pCR was highest for hormone receptor negative and HER-2 positive cancer (54%) and lowest for HR+/ Her-2 negative cancer (9%). [19], [24] In a study of 388 patients in which 16 percent patients were Her-2 positive, Her-2 positivity and young age were important predictors of achievement of pCR with anthracycline based NAC in univariate analysis. [25]

There is no single genetic marker that predicts complete response to NAC. However, gene expression profiling has been studied to predict response to various chemotherapy regimens with reasonable accuracy. [26] [27], [28] van't Veer et al developed a 70-gene expression model for prognostication using microarray analyses on 117 breast tumors. They found that genes associated with poor prognosis regulated cell cycle, metastasis, invasion and angiogenesis (eg. cyclin E2, MCM6, metalloproteinases MMP 9, MP1, RAB6B, PK428, VEGF receptor FLT1). [29] In the I SPY 1 trial, patients with p-53 null mutations and 17q amplification were also associated with high pCR rates (47% and 45% respectively). [19]

Enzymes of cytochrome P450 family play an important role in cancer drug metabolisms and polymorphism CYP2C9*2 polymorphism has been found to be associated with NAC resistance. [30] Tumor stage, lymph node positivity and dose intensity of chemotherapy have not been found to correlate to NAC response. [31] [17], [32]

Apoptotic responses to first dose of NAC measured by serial fine needle aspirations during first 4 days after chemotherapy administration was also found to be an indicator of response. [33]. Persistently elevated levels of CXCR4, a G-protein coupled receptor post chemotherapy has been found to be a negative predictor for response. [34]. A retrospective study of 562 patients concluded that metaplastic, mucinous and apocrine carcinoma responded poorly to NAC. [35]

4. Chemotherapy regimens

In the pre-taxane era, initial trials of NAC were performed with anthracycline based regimens, such as AC [3]; 5-Fluorouracil, Adriyamicin and Cyclophosphamide (FAC)[36] and 5-Fluorouracil, Epirubicin, Cyclophosphamide (FEC). [37] However, more recent trials have demonstrated that taxanes, when added to anthracycline based regimens, significantly improve survival outcomes [38] and therefore, should be used in combination with anthracycline based regimens. NSABP B-27 trial was designed to observe the impact of addition of 4 cycles of docetaxel to standard AC regimen in the preoperative setting. 2411 patients with T1C-3N0M0 or T1-3N1M0 breast tumors were assigned to ACX4 cycles vs. ACX 4 cycles followed by docetaxel X4 cycles vs. AC X 4 cycles preoperatively and docetaxel X 4 cycles postoperatively. Although the trial did not meet it's primary end point of demonstrating survival benefit, addition of docetaxel did double the pCR rates (from 13% to 26%). pCR rates were also significant predictor of improved DFS (HR: 0.49) and OS (HR: 0.36) after more than eight years of follow-up. Patients who achieved clinical partial response with AC had significantly increased DFS with addition of docetaxel [39]

For patients with the Her-2 positive cancer, trastuzumab has been incorporated in the initial neoadjuvant chemoregimens. Options include sequential trastuzumab and paclitaxel and FEC in combination with trastuzumab (PH- FECH) with pCR rates ranging from 55-65 percent. [40] However, in patients where cardiac morbidity is a concern docetaxel and cyclophosphamide in combination with trastuzumab (TCH) is also an effective choice. [41]

Capecitabine is an effective drug, which has yielded promising results in metastatic breast cancer. Capecitabine in combination of Vinorelbine has been found to be non inferior to Docetaxel, Adriyamicin, Cyclophosphamide (TAC) in terms of sonographic and pathologic complete response and breast conservation rates in the phase 3 Gepar trio trial [42]

5. Dose dense NAC

Dose intensity is achieved by increasing the drug dose delivered per cycle of chemotherapy by either increasing dose or decreasing inter-treatment interval. The PREPARE trial used dose dense (dd) and dose intensified regimens of E+ P followed by CMF and compared it with standard dose EC→T regimen. Patients were treated with E (dd) → T (250mg/m2)(dd) → CMF, each 2 weekly for 3 cycles with or without darbopoeitin versus standard E (90mg/m2) and C followed by P (150mg/m2) for four cycles (EC→T). The pCR rate was higher in the dose-dense, dose-intensified group (18.7% vs. 13.2%; p=0.04). Patients with non-inflammatory breast cancer had significantly improved disease free and overall survival from the dose dense regimens. [43]. A few other trials demonstrate similar increased in pCR rates with dose dense chemotherapy. [44] Currently, the value of dose dense chemotherapy in breast cancer is unclear amongst unselected patients.

In a phase 3 trial (SWOG 0012), standard 3 weekly AC regimen was compared to weekly doxorubicin and daily oral cyclophosphamide with GCSF support in the neoadjuvant setting for inflammatory and locally advanced breast cancer. pCR rates with the dose dense regimen were superior only in stage IIIB breast cancer and IBC. There was no difference in DFS and OS. [44]

6. Assessment of response after NAC: Definition of pCR

In most studies, pCR has been defined as absence of any residual invasive tumor in the pathologically examined tissue. Prior studies have indicated that there is no survival difference in patients with no residual tumor (in-situ or invasive) versus patients with residual in-situ (non- invasive tumor) cancer. [45] In a study performed at MD Anderson, 2302 patients treated with NAC showed similar disease free, overall and local recurrence free survival for patients who had in-situ cancer at the end of treatment when compared to patients who had no residual cancer. [46] However a recently published pooled analysis of 6,377 patients trials shows that DFS is better in patients with no residual tumor when compared to patients with residual in-situ tumor (HR:1.74, 95% CI 1.28-2.36, $p<0.001$). This study concluded that definition pCR should strictly be limited to absence of residual invasive or in-situ tumor either in the breast or lymph nodes [47].

7. Estrogen or progesterone receptor positive cancer

Although the use of endocrine therapy in the adjuvant setting is very common, it's use in the neoadjuvant setting is relatively recent. Neoadjuvant endocrine therapy has shown to cause tumor shrinkage [48] and reduce tumor proliferation as evidenced by decrease in Ki-67 and other markers of proliferation. [49] pCR is less commonly observed, therefore, response assessment in most of the trials involving endocine therapies is clinical (palpation and radiological techniques) as well as pathological assessment of proliferation markers. [50]

Comparisons have also been made between the 3 aromatase inhibitors exemestane, letrozole or anastrozole, in the neoadjuvant setting. 377 postmenopausal women with stage II/III ER positive breast cancer were treated with neoadjuvant exemestane (25mg/d), letrozole 2.5mg/d and anastrozole 1mg/d for 16-18 weeks. Clinical response rate, which was the primary end point of the trial, was 62.9%, 74.8% and 69.1% respectively. Breast conservation rates were comparable amongst the three groups. No difference was observed in terms of Ki-67 levels or changes in KI-67 expression among all the groups suggesting that they have biological equivalent effects. Overall, Luminal A tumors were likely to have a preoperative endocrine operative index (PEPI) score of zero before surgery when compared to luminal B tumors. [51]

Combination of neoadjuvant hormone and chemotherapy is also being investigated. In a phase 3 trial of 101 post menopausal women with locally advanced hormone receptor positive breast (stage T3, T4 and/ or N2 N3) cancer, neoadjuvant chemotherapy with FAC combined with letrozole 2.5mg daily produced superior pCR (25.5% VS. 10.2%, $p=0.049$) and clinical complete response rates (27.6% VS. 10.2%, $P=0.037$) when compared to FAC alone. [52]

It has been postulated that phosphotidyl kinase 3/ AKT/ mTOR pathway may be involved in endocrine resistance. For this reason, mTOR inhibitor like everolimus have been combined with hormone therapy in clinical trials. In a phase 2 trial comprising of 270 untreated patients with ER positive breast cancer, the control group was treated with letrozole (2.5mg/day) + placebo while the experimental treatment group was treated with letrozole plus everolimus (10mg/day). Patients treated with letrozole plus mTOR (mammalian target of Rapamycin) inhibitor had significantly improved clinical response rates, as well as response rates as assessed by ultrasound and mammography. Decrease in the proliferation index Ki-67 was significantly more marked with the combination treatment. Toxicities with the combination group were higher with 52.9% patients in the combination group having treatment stopped or delayed as a result of toxicities (only 7.6% in the placebo group). It was inferred that mTOR inhibitor can significantly increase the efficacy of hormone therapy. [53]

8. HER-2 receptor positive cancer

Trastuzumab or herceptin (H), a monoclonal antibody against HER-2 neu receptor, is an integral part of neoadjuvant chemotherapy in HER-2 positive tumors. In a phase 3 trial, FEC + Trastuzumab followed by P + trastuzumab has shown significantly higher pCR rates when compared to FEC→ P alone (66.7% vs. 25%). [54]

In the NeOAdjuvant herceptin (NOAH) trial, patients with HER-2 positive inflammatory or locally advanced breast cancer were treated with neoadjuvant chemotherapy alone (A+P → P→ CMF) or neoadjuvant chemotherapy combined with neoadjuvant H (added to the CMF part of neoadjuvant chemotherapy). Addition of H not only improved the rates of pathological response, (50% vs. 26%; p=0.002) but also the rates of event free survival, which was the primary end point of the study. More patients were able to undergo breast conservation surgery with the addition of H (35 vs. 13% p=0.07). [55]

Trastuzumab has been compared to lapatinib (L), a tyrosine kinase inhibitor which is a dual inhibitor of EGFR and Her-2 receptors, in the neoadjuvant setting. In the Gepar Quinto trial, patients were treated with standard chemotherapy with four cycles of Epirubicin and cyclophosphamide followed by four cycles of docetaxel along with either H (6mg/kg every 3 weeks) or L (1250mg daily) starting on the day 1 of the first EC cycle till the day 21 of the fourth cycle of docetaxel. pCR rates with H were significantly higher (30%) when compared to L (30% vs. 22%; p=0.04). Overall difference in the clinical response and the number of breast conservation surgeries between the two groups was not significant. Edema and dyspnea were more common with trastuzumab while rash and diarrhea were more common with lapatinib. [56]

Neo-Altto trial was a randomized phase 3 trial comparing dual (trastuzumab/lapatinib combination) versus single Her-2 receptor blockade (trastuzumab or lapatinib alone) for HER-2 positive breast cancer, >2cm in diameter along with a taxane in the neoadjuvant setting. 154 patients received 1500mg of PO lapatinib, 149 received 4mg IV trastuzumab (2mg/kg subsequent doses) and 152 received the combination of trastuzumab with 1000mg PO lapatinib. pCR rates were significantly higher with dual blockade (51.3 percent; 95% C.I.

43.1-59.5%) when compared to single blockade with trastuzumab alone (29.5%; 95% C.I. 22.4-37.5). No significant difference in the pCR rates between trastuzumab and lapatinib groups was observed (p=0.34). Grade 3 diarrhea and elevation of liver enzymes were more common side effects in the lapatinib (23.4%) and lapatinib plus trastuzumab group (21.1%) when compared to trastuzumab only group (2%). The rate of breast conservation surgery in all the three groups was similar. pCR rate was higher in the ER negative tumors. [57]

In the preliminary results of the NSABP B-41 trial presented in American Society of Clinical Oncology's (ASCO) annual meeting in 2012, when H is substituted with L, the responses pCR rates are found to be comparable. This trial comparing AC→ weekly paclitaxel (WP)+ H vs. AC→ WP + L vs. AC→ WP+ H+L; showed that pCR rates with H and L were comparable (52.5% for T vs. 53.2% for L). pCR rates with the combination of both T and L with NAC was slightly higher but the results were not statistically significant (62% p= 0.075). [58]

Trastuzumab has been combined with another humanized monoclonal antibody against HER-2, Pertuzumab, which binds the dimerization site of HER-2 receptor and inhibits ligand dependent signaling. The phase 2 multicenter Neosphere trial compared combinations of H+ T (group A), H+ Pertuzumab +T (group B), Pertuzumab +H (group C) and pertuzumab + T (group D) as neoadjuvant treatment of Her-2 positive breast cancer. The pCR rates in group B was significantly higher (45.8%, p=0.0141) when compared to groups A, C or D (29%, 16.8% and 24 % respectively). Clinical responses to NAC were also highest in group B. The rate of febrile neutropenia was similar in the trastuzumab+ pertuzumab + chemotherapy group to the H+ T group and was 7-8%. [59]

Trastuzumab combined with bevacizumab and chemotherapy was found to be very effective in Her-2 positive inflammatory breast cancer in the phase 2 BEVERLY-2 trial. In this study, 52 patients were treated with FEC + Bevacizumab (cycles 1-4) and docetaxel +bevacizumab and trastuzumab (cycles 5-8). pCR was seen in 33 patients (63.5%). The frequency of grade ¾ neutropenia was 48%. [60]

9. Role of bevacizumab

Bevacizumab is a monoclonal antibody against vascular endothelial growth factor (VEGF), which has been found to be very effective when added to anthracycline- taxane based neoadjuvant therapy. In the phase 3 NSABP- 40 trial, [61] patients with T1c-T3/ N0-N2 were treated with the following regimens: Docetaxel (T) alone followed by EC vs. T + Gemcitabine followed by EC vs. T + G + Bevacizumab followed by EC vs. T + Capecitabine (X) followed by EC vs. T + X + Bevacizumab followed by EC. Addition of bevacizumab significantly increased the pCR rates in the breast, which was the primary end point of this study (28.2% to 34.5%, p=0.02). pCR rate in breast and nodes (secondary end point) was also increased but the result was not significant. Rate of clinical complete responses was significantly increased with addition of bevacizumab. Effect of bevacizumab was more pronounced in hormone receptor positive tumor and higher tumor grade. Side effects observed with bevacizumab included significantly higher rates of hypertension, left ventricular systolic dysfunction, mucositis and hand-foot syndrome.

Another phase 3 trial (GEPAR QUITNO) consisting if 1948 HER-2 negative patients concluded that rates of pCR were significantly improved when bevacizumab was added to EC→ T regimen (14.9% with EC→T alone and 18.4% with EC→ T+ Bevacizumab). In this study, improvement in pCR was limited to patients with hormone receptor negative tumor (39 with beviciz umab VS. 28% without bevacizumab). Side effect profile of bevacizumab was similar to the abovementioned study. [62]

Findings of the above two studies have led to conflicting results. While former has shown benefit of bevacizumab in hormone receptor positive patients, the latter has shown benefit in hormone negative cancer. A phase 3 ARTemis trial is currently underway which compares addition of bevacizumab to standard chemotherapy to chemotherapy alone. The study is to finish recruitment in December 2012 and primary outcome analysis due by December 2013. [63]

However, in some other trials, addition of bevacizumab to chemotherapy has shown less efficacy with additional toxicity. In one study, 45 women with Her2 negative locally advanced breast cancer were treated with neoadjuvant AC + bevacizumab X4 cycles followed by TX+ bevacizumab X4 cycles, with pCR rates of only 9 percent with substantial added toxicity such as fatigue, mucositis and headache. [64]

Trials looking at pathological markers predicting response to bevacizumab have shown positive responses associated with negative hormone receptor status, high Ki67 index and changes in phosphorilation status of VEGF receptor 2 (
J Clin Oncol 30, 2012 (suppl; abstr 10595))

10. NAC in triple negative breast cancer

Triple negative breast cancer is a more aggressive form of breast cancer that has poor prognosis despite response to chemotherapy. TNBC has been found to be sensitive to platinum based treatment in the metastatic setting due to inherent genomic instability. Encouraged by success in the metastatic setting, trials have been conducted with platinum agents in the primary setting. Silver et al. treated 28 patients with stage II/III TNBC with four three weekly cycles of cisplatin. pCR was seen in 22% patients; good pathological response (Miller Payne score of 3,4 or 5) in 50% and progression in 14% patients. Positive response to cisplatin in this study was associated with young age, low BRCA expression, BRCA-1 prominent methylation, p-53 frameshift or nonsense mutation and gene expression significant of E2F3 activation. [65] More pCR rates have been demonstrated in BRCA-1 mutated breast cancers with cisplatin than with conventional regimens such as AC or CMF. [66] In another study, 17 patients with triple negative breast cancers >2cm in size, were treated with weekly doxorubicin plus daily oral cyclphosphamide followed by weekly paclitaxel and carboplatin, 14 out of 15 assessable patients showed clinical response. pCR rate was 46.6%. Seven patients had grade ¾ hematological toxicity with this combination. [67] Similar high pCR rates have been reported with neoadjuvant bevacizumab, docetaxel and Carboplatin combination. [68] However, in a multicenter phase 2 study, addition of carboplatin to standard EC→T regimen for basal like breast cancer (defined as ER-/PR-/Her2-/Cytokeratin 5/6+ and /or EGFR+) did not enhance efficacy of standard chemotherapy (pCR rates: 35% vs. 30% in Carboplatin vs. no Carboplatin group, p=0.6064). [69]

The phase 3 GeparQuinto study demonstrated that addition of Bevacizumab to conventional chemotherapy (EC→ T) can further improve pathological CR (pCR) rates in triple negative breast cancer. [62]. However, as mentioned above, these findings contradict with the NSABP B40 study where major benefit was obtained in hormone positive cancer. [70] Carboplatin in combination with weekly nab paclitaxel and bevacizumab is also currently being evaluated in a clinical study. [71]

Ixabepilone is a new class of semisynthetic microtubule inhibiting drugs which is derived from natural epithilones. It has shown promising results in metastatic and multidrug resistant (anthracyclines, capecitabine, taxanes) breast cancer. [72]- [76] In a phase 2 study designed to assess benefit of ixabepilone in the neoadjuvant setting, 161 patients were treated with four cycles of ixabepilone. pCR was observed in 18% in all patients, but in 29% of ER negative patients, ER gene expression was inversely related to response in this study. [77] A pooled analysis of data from five phase 2 and two phase 3 trials, pCR rates with ixabepilone in the neoadjuvant setting were 26% in TNBC vs. 15% in non TNBC. [77], [78] Newer non-taxane microtubule inhibiting agents such as eribulin are being evaluated as NAC for TNBC in clinical trials.

Poly ADP ribose polymerase (PARP) inhibitors inhibit the PARP-1 enzyme which is a DNA base excision repair enzyme and along with BRCA, is involved in cell's DNA repair. [79], [80] It's role in tumorigenesis in evidenced by it's upregulation seen in tumor cells, thus protecting cancer cell DNA from damage and cell death. [81] PARP inhibition leads to cell death by two mechanisms. First, it causes accumulation of single and double stranded DNA breaks causing subsequent cell death. Secondly, it causes sensitization to therapeutic DNA damage. [82] Two trials utilizing PARP inhibitor Iniparib in combination of preoperative setting are underway and results are expected soon.

11. Role of neoadjuvant chemoradiation

In a multi-institutional study, 105 patients with locally advanced breast cancer were treated with twice weekly paclitaxel 30mg/m2 for 10-12 weeks and radiation therapy (total 45gy) over weeks 2-7. Trastuzumab was added to this regimen in patients found to be Her-2 positive. Pathological response (complete and partial) was achieved in 34% patients and was found to be significantly higher in hormone receptor negative patients (54%, 95% C.I. 36%-69%) and triple negative tumors (54%). As expected, patients who achieved pathological response had higher disease free survival (57 months vs. not reached, HR: 2.85, p<0.001) and overall survival (84 months vs. not reached, HR: 4.27). [83]

http://dx.doi.org/10.5772/53192

12. Monitoring response to NAC

Assessment of radiological response especially when using MRI or PET scan is very useful since it may help in early differentiation of responders to NAC from non-responders.

Studies have shown that decrease in tumor volume and enhancement on contrast enhanced MRI is associated with major histopathological response. [84], [85] Loo et al showed that MRI was able to monitor response to NAC more accurately in TNBC and Her-2 positive subsets but not in ER+, Her-2 negative subsets. [86] The I-SPY-1 study found that decrease in tumor volume as assessed by MRI early during treatment with NAC was a better predictor of pathologic response than measurement of tumor diameter by physical examination alone.

PET CT is another valuable imaging modality for accurately predicting response to NAC early in the course if therapy. [87], [88] In a study of 33 patients treated with carboplatin based NAC, there was significant correlation between FDG PET metabolic response after first and third cycles and overall survival. [89]

Studies have compared MRI and PET scan as predictors of response to NAC. Choi et al found that compared to PET CT, MRI was highly predictive of pCR ($P<0.005$) and better than PET CT for monitoring response to NAC. [90] However, Rousseau et al found that using 60% cut off value for SUV, the sensitivity, specificity and negative predictive value of PET scan were 89%, 955 and 85% respectively after two cycles of NAC. Values were much lower for US and mammography. Tateishi et al also found PET CT to be superior to DCE MRI for pCR prediction after 2 cycles of NAC. [91]

13. Conclusion

NAC is the standard of care in management of locally advanced and inoperable breast cancer. It significantly downstages the tumor, thereby permitting breast conservation surgery. Anthracycline and taxanes based regimens are most commonly used NAC regimens. For Her-2 positive tumors, trastuzumab should be included in the NAC regimen. Role of other targeted therapies in NAC is being investigated.

Author details

Jasmeet Chadha Singh and Amy Tiersten

New York University Medical Center, New York, NY, USA, USA

References

[1] Chollet P, Amat S, Cure H, et al: Prognostic significance of a complete pathological response after induction chemotherapy in operable breast cancer. Br J Cancer 86:1041-6, 2002

[2] Rastogi P, Anderson SJ, Bear HD, et al: Preoperative chemotherapy: updates of National Surgical Adjuvant Breast and Bowel Project Protocols B-18 and B-27. J Clin Oncol 26:778-85, 2008

[3] Wolmark N, Wang J, Mamounas E, et al: Preoperative chemotherapy in patients with operable breast cancer: nine-year results from National Surgical Adjuvant Breast and Bowel Project B-18. J Natl Cancer Inst Monogr:96-102, 2001

[4] Bear HD, Anderson S, Smith RE, et al: Sequential preoperative or postoperative docetaxel added to preoperative doxorubicin plus cyclophosphamide for operable breast cancer:National Surgical Adjuvant Breast and Bowel Project Protocol B-27. J Clin Oncol 24:2019-27, 2006

[5] Kuerer HM, Newman LA, Smith TL, et al: Clinical course of breast cancer patients with complete pathologic primary tumor and axillary lymph node response to doxorubicin-based neoadjuvant chemotherapy. J Clin Oncol 17:460-9, 1999

[6] Zhang GC, Qian XK, Guo ZB, et al: Pre-treatment hormonal receptor status and Ki67 index predict pathologic complete response to neoadjuvant trastuzumab/taxanes but not disease-free survival in HER2-positive breast cancer patients. Med Oncol, 2012

[7] Liedtke C, Mazouni C, Hess KR, et al: Response to neoadjuvant therapy and long-term survival in patients with triple-negative breast cancer. J Clin Oncol 26:1275-81, 2008

[8] Carey LA, Dees EC, Sawyer L, et al: The triple negative paradox: primary tumor chemosensitivity of breast cancer subtypes. Clin Cancer Res 13:2329-34, 2007

[9] Esserman LJ, Berry DA, Demichele A, et al: Pathologic Complete Response Predicts Recurrence-Free Survival More Effectively by Cancer Subset: Results From the I-SPY 1 TRIAL--CALGB 150007/150012, ACRIN 6657. J Clin Oncol, 2012

[10] Untch M, Fasching PA, Konecny GE, et al: Pathologic complete response after neoadjuvant chemotherapy plus trastuzumab predicts favorable survival in human epidermal growth factor receptor 2-overexpressing breast cancer: results from the TECHNO trial of the AGO and GBG study groups. J Clin Oncol 29:3351-7, 2011

[11] Gianni L, Baselga J, Eiermann W, et al: Phase III trial evaluating the addition of paclitaxel to doxorubicin followed by cyclophosphamide, methotrexate, and fluorouracil, as adjuvant or primary systemic therapy: European Cooperative Trial in Operable Breast Cancer. J Clin Oncol 27:2474-81, 2009

[12] Andre F, Mazouni C, Liedtke C, et al: HER2 expression and efficacy of preoperative paclitaxel/FAC chemotherapy in breast cancer. Breast Cancer Res Treat 108:183-90, 2008

[13] Osako T, Horii R, Matsuura M, et al: High-grade breast cancers include both highly sensitive and highly resistant subsets to cytotoxic chemotherapy. J Cancer Res Clin Oncol 136:1431-8, 2010

[14] Fisher ER, Wang J, Bryant J, et al: Pathobiology of preoperative chemotherapy: findings from the National Surgical Adjuvant Breast and Bowel (NSABP) protocol B-18. Cancer 95:681-95, 2002

[15] Horii R, Akiyama F, Ito Y, et al: Histological features of breast cancer, highly sensitive to chemotherapy. Breast Cancer 14:393-400, 2007

[16] Rouzier R, Pusztai L, Delaloge S, et al: Nomograms to predict pathologic complete response and metastasis-free survival after preoperative chemotherapy for breast cancer. J Clin Oncol 23:8331-9, 2005

[17] Wang J, Buchholz TA, Middleton LP, et al: Assessment of histologic features and expression of biomarkers in predicting pathologic response to anthracycline-based neoadjuvant chemotherapy in patients with breast carcinoma. Cancer 94:3107-14, 2002

[18] Sanchez-Rovira P, Anton A, Barnadas A, et al: Classical markers like ER and ki-67, but also survivin and pERK, could be involved in the pathological response to gemcitabine, adriamycin and paclitaxel (GAT) in locally advanced breast cancer patients: results from the GEICAM/2002-01 phase II study. Clin Transl Oncol 14:430-6, 2012

[19] Esserman LJ, Berry DA, Cheang MC, et al: Chemotherapy response and recurrence-free survival in neoadjuvant breast cancer depends on biomarker profiles: results from the I-SPY 1 TRIAL (CALGB 150007/150012; ACRIN 6657). Breast Cancer Res Treat 132:1049-62, 2012

[20] al. Ae: Role of proliferation in response to neoadjuvant chemotherapy in GEICAM/2006-03 and GEICAM/2006-14 breast cancer patients. J Clin Oncol, 2012

[21] Rouzier R, Perou CM, Symmans WF, et al: Breast cancer molecular subtypes respond differently to preoperative chemotherapy. Clin Cancer Res 11:5678-85, 2005

[22] Li XR, Liu M, Zhang YJ, et al: CK5/6, EGFR, Ki-67, cyclin D1, and nm23-H1 protein expressions as predictors of pathological complete response to neoadjuvant chemotherapy in triple-negative breast cancer patients. Med Oncol 28 Suppl 1:S129-34, 2011

[23] Keam B, Im SA, Kim HJ, et al: Prognostic impact of clinicopathologic parameters in stage II/III breast cancer treated with neoadjuvant docetaxel and doxorubicin chemotherapy: paradoxical features of the triple negative breast cancer. BMC Cancer 7:203, 2007

[24] Li XR, Liu M, Zhang YJ, et al: ER, PgR, HER-2, Ki-67, topoisomerase IIalpha, and nm23-H1 proteins expression as predictors of pathological complete response to neo-

adjuvant chemotherapy for locally advanced breast cancer. Med Oncol 28 Suppl 1:S48-54, 2011

[25] Keskin S, Muslumanoglu M, Saip P, et al: Clinical and pathological features of breast cancer associated with the pathological complete response to anthracycline-based neoadjuvant chemotherapy. Oncology 81:30-8, 2011

[26] Dejeux E, Ronneberg JA, Solvang H, et al: DNA methylation profiling in doxorubicin treated primary locally advanced breast tumours identifies novel genes associated with survival and treatment response. Mol Cancer 9:68, 2010

[27] Ayers M, Symmans WF, Stec J, et al: Gene expression profiles predict complete pathologic response to neoadjuvant paclitaxel and fluorouracil, doxorubicin, and cyclophosphamide chemotherapy in breast cancer. J Clin Oncol 22:2284-93, 2004

[28] Zembutsu H, Suzuki Y, Sasaki A, et al: Predicting response to docetaxel neoadjuvant chemotherapy for advanced breast cancers through genome-wide gene expression profiling. Int J Oncol 34:361-70, 2009

[29] van 't Veer LJ, Dai H, van de Vijver MJ, et al: Gene expression profiling predicts clinical outcome of breast cancer. Nature 415:530-6, 2002

[30] Seredina TA, Goreva OB, Talaban VO, et al: Association of cytochrome P450 genetic polymorphisms with neoadjuvant chemotherapy efficacy in breast cancer patients. BMC Med Genet 13:45, 2012

[31] Huober J, von Minckwitz G, Denkert C, et al: Effect of neoadjuvant anthracycline-taxane-based chemotherapy in different biological breast cancer phenotypes: overall results from the GeparTrio study. Breast Cancer Res Treat 124:133-40, 2010

[32] Iwase S, Yamamoto D, Kuroda Y, et al: Phase II trial of preoperative chemotherapy for breast cancer: Japan Breast Cancer Research Network (JBCRN)-02 trial. Anticancer Res 31:1483-7, 2011

[33] Symmans WF, Volm MD, Shapiro RL, et al: Paclitaxel-induced apoptosis and mitotic arrest assessed by serial fine-needle aspiration: implications for early prediction of breast cancer response to neoadjuvant treatment. Clin Cancer Res 6:4610-7, 2000

[34] Hiller DJ, Li BD, Chu QD: CXCR4 as a predictive marker for locally advanced breast cancer post-neoadjuvant therapy. J Surg Res 166:14-8, 2011

[35] Nagao T, Kinoshita T, Hojo T, et al: The differences in the histological types of breast cancer and the response to neoadjuvant chemotherapy: The relationship between the outcome and the clinicopathological characteristics. Breast 21:289-95, 2012

[36] Hortobagyi GN, Ames FC, Buzdar AU, et al: Management of stage III primary breast cancer with primary chemotherapy, surgery, and radiation therapy. Cancer 62:2507-16, 1988

[37] van der Hage JA, van de Velde CJ, Julien JP, et al: Preoperative chemotherapy in primary operable breast cancer: results from the European Organization for Research and Treatment of Cancer trial 10902. J Clin Oncol 19:4224-37, 2001

[38] Buzdar AU, Singletary SE, Theriault RL, et al: Prospective evaluation of paclitaxel versus combination chemotherapy with fluorouracil, doxorubicin, and cyclophosphamide as neoadjuvant therapy in patients with operable breast cancer. J Clin Oncol 17:3412-7, 1999

[39] Bear HD, Anderson S, Brown A, et al: The effect on tumor response of adding sequential preoperative docetaxel to preoperative doxorubicin and cyclophosphamide: preliminary results from National Surgical Adjuvant Breast and Bowel Project Protocol B-27. J Clin Oncol 21:4165-74, 2003

[40] Buzdar AU, Valero V, Ibrahim NK, et al: Neoadjuvant therapy with paclitaxel followed by 5-fluorouracil, epirubicin, and cyclophosphamide chemotherapy and concurrent trastuzumab in human epidermal growth factor receptor 2-positive operable breast cancer: an update of the initial randomized study population and data of additional patients treated with the same regimen. Clin Cancer Res 13:228-33, 2007

[41] Chang H: Clinical Advantages of Neoadjuvant Docetaxel (T) and Carboplatin (C) ± Trastuzumab (H) in Locally Advanced Breast Cancer (LABC). Cancer Research 69, 2009

[42] von Minckwitz G, Kummel S, Vogel P, et al: Neoadjuvant vinorelbine-capecitabine versus docetaxel-doxorubicin-cyclophosphamide in early nonresponsive breast cancer: phase III randomized GeparTrio trial. J Natl Cancer Inst 100:542-51, 2008

[43] Untch M, Fasching PA, Konecny GE, et al: PREPARE trial: a randomized phase III trial comparing preoperative, dose-dense, dose-intensified chemotherapy with epirubicin, paclitaxel and CMF versus a standard-dosed epirubicin/cyclophosphamide followed by paclitaxel +/- darbepoetin alfa in primary breast cancer--results at the time of surgery. Ann Oncol 22:1988-98, 2011

[44] Ellis GK, Barlow WE, Gralow JR, et al: Phase III comparison of standard doxorubicin and cyclophosphamide versus weekly doxorubicin and daily oral cyclophosphamide plus granulocyte colony-stimulating factor as neoadjuvant therapy for inflammatory and locally advanced breast cancer: SWOG 0012. J Clin Oncol 29:1014-21, 2011

[45] Jones RL, Lakhani SR, Ring AE, et al: Pathological complete response and residual DCIS following neoadjuvant chemotherapy for breast carcinoma. Br J Cancer 94:358-62, 2006

[46] Mazouni C, Peintinger F, Wan-Kau S, et al: Residual ductal carcinoma in situ in patients with complete eradication of invasive breast cancer after neoadjuvant chemotherapy does not adversely affect patient outcome. J Clin Oncol 25:2650-5, 2007

[47] von Minckwitz G, Untch M, Blohmer JU, et al: Definition and impact of pathologic complete response on prognosis after neoadjuvant chemotherapy in various intrinsic breast cancer subtypes. J Clin Oncol 30:1796-804, 2012

[48] Dixon JM, Renshaw L, Bellamy C, et al: The effects of neoadjuvant anastrozole (Arimidex) on tumor volume in postmenopausal women with breast cancer: a randomized, double-blind, single-center study. Clin Cancer Res 6:2229-35, 2000

[49] Anderson TJ, Dixon JM, Stuart M, et al: Effect of neoadjuvant treatment with anastrozole on tumour histology in postmenopausal women with large operable breast cancer. Br J Cancer 87:334-8, 2002

[50] Dowsett M, Ebbs SR, Dixon JM, et al: Biomarker changes during neoadjuvant anastrozole, tamoxifen, or the combination: influence of hormonal status and HER-2 in breast cancer--a study from the IMPACT trialists. J Clin Oncol 23:2477-92, 2005

[51] Ellis MJ, Suman VJ, Hoog J, et al: Randomized phase II neoadjuvant comparison between letrozole, anastrozole, and exemestane for postmenopausal women with estrogen receptor-rich stage 2 to 3 breast cancer: clinical and biomarker outcomes and predictive value of the baseline PAM50-based intrinsic subtype--ACOSOG Z1031. J Clin Oncol 29:2342-9, 2011

[52] Mohammadianpanah M, Ashouri Y, Hoseini S, et al: The efficacy and safety of neoadjuvant chemotherapy +/- letrozole in postmenopausal women with locally advanced breast cancer: a randomized phase III clinical trial. Breast Cancer Res Treat 132:853-61, 2012

[53] Baselga J, Semiglazov V, van Dam P, et al: Phase II randomized study of neoadjuvant everolimus plus letrozole compared with placebo plus letrozole in patients with estrogen receptor-positive breast cancer. J Clin Oncol 27:2630-7, 2009

[54] Buzdar AU, Ibrahim NK, Francis D, et al: Significantly higher pathologic complete remission rate after neoadjuvant therapy with trastuzumab, paclitaxel, and epirubicin chemotherapy: results of a randomized trial in human epidermal growth factor receptor 2-positive operable breast cancer. J Clin Oncol 23:3676-85, 2005

[55] Semiglazov V, Eiermann W, Zambetti M, et al: Surgery following neoadjuvant therapy in patients with HER2-positive locally advanced or inflammatory breast cancer participating in the NeOAdjuvant Herceptin (NOAH) study. Eur J Surg Oncol 37:856-63, 2011

[56] Untch M, Loibl S, Bischoff J, et al: Lapatinib versus trastuzumab in combination with neoadjuvant anthracycline-taxane-based chemotherapy (GeparQuinto, GBG 44): a randomised phase 3 trial. Lancet Oncol 13:135-44, 2012

[57] Baselga J, Bradbury I, Eidtmann H, et al: Lapatinib with trastuzumab for HER2-positive early breast cancer (NeoALTTO): a randomised, open-label, multicentre, phase 3 trial. Lancet 379:633-40, 2012

[58] al Re: Evaluation of lapatinib as a component of neoadjuvant therapy for HER2+ operable breast cancer: NSABP protocol B-41. J Clin Oncol, 2012

[59] Gianni L, Pienkowski T, Im YH, et al: Efficacy and safety of neoadjuvant pertuzumab and trastuzumab in women with locally advanced, inflammatory, or early HER2-positive breast cancer (NeoSphere): a randomised multicentre, open-label, phase 2 trial. Lancet Oncol 13:25-32, 2012

[60] Pierga JY, Petit T, Delozier T, et al: Neoadjuvant bevacizumab, trastuzumab, and chemotherapy for primary inflammatory HER2-positive breast cancer (BEVERLY-2): an open-label, single-arm phase 2 study. Lancet Oncol 13:375-84, 2012

[61] Bear HD, Tang G, Rastogi P, et al: Bevacizumab added to neoadjuvant chemotherapy for breast cancer. N Engl J Med 366:310-20, 2012

[62] von Minckwitz G, Eidtmann H, Rezai M, et al: Neoadjuvant chemotherapy and bevacizumab for HER2-negative breast cancer. N Engl J Med 366:299-309, 2012

[63] al. Ee: ARTemis: Randomized trial with neoadjuvant chemotherapy for patients with early breast cancer. J Clin Oncol, 2012

[64] Rastogi P, Buyse ME, Swain SM, et al: Concurrent bevacizumab with a sequential regimen of doxorubicin and cyclophosphamide followed by docetaxel and capecitabine as neoadjuvant therapy for HER2- locally advanced breast cancer: a phase II trial of the NSABP Foundation Research Group. Clin Breast Cancer 11:228-34, 2011

[65] Silver DP, Richardson AL, Eklund AC, et al: Efficacy of neoadjuvant Cisplatin in triple-negative breast cancer. J Clin Oncol 28:1145-53, 2010

[66] Byrski T, Gronwald J, Huzarski T, et al: Pathologic complete response rates in young women with BRCA1-positive breast cancers after neoadjuvant chemotherapy. J Clin Oncol 28:375-9, 2010

[67] al. Te: Results of the East Carolina Breast Center phase II trial of neoadjuvant metronomic chemotherapy in triple-negative breast cancer (NCT00542191). J Clin Oncol, 2012

[68] al. Ke: A multicenter phase II neoadjuvant trial of bevacizumab combined with docetaxel plus carboplatin in the treatment of triple-negative breast cancer: Korean Cancer Study Group (KCSG-BR 0905, NCT 01208480). J Clin Oncol, 2012

[69] al. EAe: Chemotherapy (CT) with or without carboplatin as neoadjuvant treatment in patients with basal-like breast cancer: GEICAM 2006-03-A multicenter, randomized phase II study. J Clin Oncol 29, 2011

[70] al. Be: Phase II neoadjuvant trial with carboplatin and eribulin mesylate in patients with triple-negative breast cancer. J Clin Oncol, 2012

[71] al. Se: Neoadjuvant bevacizumab with weekly nab-paclitaxel plus carboplatin followed by doxorubicin plus cyclophosphamide (AC) for triple-negative breast cancer. J Clin Oncol, 2012

[72] Roche H, Yelle L, Cognetti F, et al: Phase II clinical trial of ixabepilone (BMS-247550), an epothilone B analog, as first-line therapy in patients with metastatic breast cancer previously treated with anthracycline chemotherapy. J Clin Oncol 25:3415-20, 2007

[73] Low JA, Wedam SB, Lee JJ, et al: Phase II clinical trial of ixabepilone (BMS-247550), an epothilone B analog, in metastatic and locally advanced breast cancer. J Clin Oncol 23:2726-34, 2005

[74] Perez EA, Lerzo G, Pivot X, et al: Efficacy and safety of ixabepilone (BMS-247550) in a phase II study of patients with advanced breast cancer resistant to an anthracycline, a taxane, and capecitabine. J Clin Oncol 25:3407-14, 2007

[75] Thomas E, Tabernero J, Fornier M, et al: Phase II clinical trial of ixabepilone (BMS-247550), an epothilone B analog, in patients with taxane-resistant metastatic breast cancer. J Clin Oncol 25:3399-406, 2007

[76] Thomas ES, Gomez HL, Li RK, et al: Ixabepilone plus capecitabine for metastatic breast cancer progressing after anthracycline and taxane treatment. J Clin Oncol 25:5210-7, 2007

[77] Baselga J, Zambetti M, Llombart-Cussac A, et al: Phase II genomics study of ixabepilone as neoadjuvant treatment for breast cancer. J Clin Oncol 27:526-34, 2009

[78] Perez EA, Patel T, Moreno-Aspitia A: Efficacy of ixabepilone in ER/PR/HER2-negative (triple-negative) breast cancer. Breast Cancer Res Treat 121:261-71, 2010

[79] Hanahan D, Weinberg RA: Hallmarks of cancer: the next generation. Cell 144:646-74, 2011

[80] Harper JW, Elledge SJ: The DNA damage response: ten years after. Mol Cell 28:739-45, 2007

[81] Ossovskaya V, Koo IC, Kaldjian EP, et al: Upregulation of Poly (ADP-Ribose) Polymerase-1 (PARP1) in Triple-Negative Breast Cancer and Other Primary Human Tumor Types. Genes Cancer 1:812-21, 2010

[82] Farmer H, McCabe N, Lord CJ, et al: Targeting the DNA repair defect in BRCA mutant cells as a therapeutic strategy. Nature 434:917-21, 2005

[83] Adams S, Chakravarthy AB, Donach M, et al: Preoperative concurrent paclitaxel-radiation in locally advanced breast cancer: pathologic response correlates with five-year overall survival. Breast Cancer Res Treat 124:723-32, 2010

[84] Martincich L, Montemurro F, De Rosa G, et al: Monitoring response to primary chemotherapy in breast cancer using dynamic contrast-enhanced magnetic resonance imaging. Breast Cancer Res Treat 83:67-76, 2004

[85] Hylton NM, Blume JD, Bernreuter WK, et al: Locally Advanced Breast Cancer: MR Imaging for Prediction of Response to Neoadjuvant Chemotherapy--Results from ACRIN 6657/I-SPY TRIAL. Radiology 263:663-672, 2012

[86] Loo CE, Straver ME, Rodenhuis S, et al: Magnetic resonance imaging response monitoring of breast cancer during neoadjuvant chemotherapy: relevance of breast cancer subtype. J Clin Oncol 29:660-6, 2011

[87] Inokuchi M, Furukawa H, Kayahara M, et al: [The role of / 18FDG PET/CT for the initial staging and therapy in primary breast cancer]. Gan To Kagaku Ryoho 36:2526-31, 2009

[88] Schelling M, Avril N, Nahrig J, et al: Positron emission tomography using [(18)F]Fluorodeoxyglucose for monitoring primary chemotherapy in breast cancer. J Clin Oncol 18:1689-95, 2000

[89] Avril N, Sassen S, Schmalfeldt B, et al: Prediction of response to neoadjuvant chemotherapy by sequential F-18-fluorodeoxyglucose positron emission tomography in patients with advanced-stage ovarian cancer. J Clin Oncol 23:7445-53, 2005

[90] Choi JH, Lim HI, Lee SK, et al: The role of PET CT to evaluate the response to neoadjuvant chemotherapy in advanced breast cancer: comparison with ultrasonography and magnetic resonance imaging. J Surg Oncol 102:392-7, 2010

[91] Tateishi U, Miyake M, Nagaoka T, et al: Neoadjuvant chemotherapy in breast cancer: prediction of pathologic response with PET/CT and dynamic contrast-enhanced MR imaging--prospective assessment. Radiology 263:53-63, 2012

Section 2

Neoadjuvant Chemotherapy of Other Malignancies

Chapter 5

Rationale for Neoadjuvant Chemotherapy in the Management of Malignant Disease

Maurie Markman

Additional information is available at the end of the chapter

http://dx.doi.org/10.5772/55393

1. Introduction

In the earliest days of the modern anti-neoplastic chemotherapeutic era the focus of such therapy in solid tumor oncology was on the management of recurrent or metastatic cancer. Over the past several decades the outcomes of such treatment, both an improvement in survival and a reduction in the toxicities associated with this strategy have made some form of drug therapy routine care in most advanced human malignancies.

Subsequent efforts demonstrated the effectiveness associated with the administration of anti-neoplastic agents in the *adjuvant setting* prior to the documentation of the existence of metastatic cancer. Such therapy was justified where there was a recognized known unacceptable risk that the disease may still be present within the individual patient despite appropriate local therapy (e.g., surgery, radiation therapy, or both).

2. Rationale for neoadjuvant chemotherapy in the management of malignant disease

The concept of *neoadjuvant chemotherapy* is a newer addition to the anti-neoplastic drug strategies employed in routine cancer management. The several important and unique goals associated with this approach in contrast to chemotherapy delivered as adjuvant therapy or as treatment of metastatic disease are outlined in Table 1.

It is reasonable to suggest the initial use of the therapeutic concept of neoadjuvant therapy developed in settings where individual oncologists believed local disease control would simply not be able to be achieved due to the extent of local tumor (e.g., large locally-advanced breast, bladder or esophageal cancer), where the signs/symptoms of the cancer increased the risks associated with attempting to accomplish this goal (e.g., rapidly accumulating ascites in a patient with extensive intra-abdominal carcinomatosis from ovarian cancer), or when existing co-morbidity precluded consideration of such surgery (e.g., recent history of myocardial ischemia).

However, in recent years investigators have begun to speculate that rather than simply being a reluctantly delivered less effective alternative, the successful use of an initial neoadjuvant approach (chemotherapy alone or combined with external beam radiation) may actually permit the subsequent undertaking of definitive local/regional treatment to a substantially larger percentage of patients who present with a particular clinical scenario [1-7].

Thus, the advanced ovarian cancer patient with extensive intra-abdominal cancer who would have required a very extensive operation of quite uncertain value performed at a time of nutritional/protein depletion (secondary to massive fluid present within the peritoneal cavity in addition to poor appetite) may be able to successfully undergo surgery to remove all visible cancer following the administration of chemotherapy that substantially reduces tumor volume. In fact, a published landmark phase 3 randomized trial has now confirmed that the administration of neoadjuvant chemotherapy (carboplatin plus paclitaxel) in this exact clinical setting not only results in an identical overall survival outcome, compared to primary surgery in women with advanced ovarian cancer, but actually accomplishes this goal with less morbidity and surgery-associated mortality [4].

And in the setting of locally advanced breast cancer the administration of neoadjuvant chemotherapy designed to reduce the extent of tumor involvement may permit disease control in this region to be achieved without the requirement for a cosmetically unacceptable outcome (due to the extent of the otherwise necessary surgery) [6,7].

A particularly attractive feature of the concept of neoadjuvant chemotherapy is the ability to define the inherent chemosensitivity of an individual cancer *in vivo* within a particular patient. In certain clinical settings where the biological activity of available chemotherapy is unfortunately anticipated to be quite modest (at best), knowledge that the specific cancer has decreased in size prior to surgical resection can be one critically relevant component in the decision to continue adjuvant therapy with the same drug(s) in that individual.

Similarly, the failure of a neoadjuvant chemotherapy regimen to produce the anticipated biological and clinical outcome in a particular patient (e.g., advanced ovarian cancer with an objective response rate of 70-80%) should result in very serious questions being raised about the wisdom of continuing with the original plan to subject the patient to an attempt at maximal surgical cytoreduction. In fact, if the patient has failed to respond to the best chemotherapy available when delivered in the neoadjuvant setting, it is most difficult to see the benefits of surgery considering the very small changes a second line chemotherapy approach will have a favorable impact on the course of the illness. It should be noted that in some circumstances surgical intervention for the specific purpose of providing palliation of distressing cancer-related symptoms may still be considered appropriate in carefully selected patients even if definitive surgical resection is realistically no longer a viable therapeutic option.

http://dx.doi.org/10.5772/55393

With increasing evidence supporting a role of molecular testing in the selection of an optimal management strategy one could envision a novel role for the neoadjuvant therapy strategy. Following the performance of such testing, the selection of a novel treatment and the observation of an outcome (e.g., tumor regression, progression), the *re-biopsy and re-analysis of changes in the molecular profile of the residual cancer might help inform decisions regarding future therapy*. It is reasonable to anticipate that there will be considerable clinical cancer research undertaken in the future that employs this basic paradigm. Finally, it is not unreasonable to anticipate that this approach will someday become a component of standard-of-care medical management in some malignancies.

1. Reduce the risk of serious treatment-related morbidity or treatment-related mortality associated with attempting to achieve definitive local disease control
2. Enhance the chances definitive local disease control will be associated with an optimal quality-of-life outcome
3. Increase the proportion of patients in a particular clinical setting who will be candidates to undergo a realistic attempt to achieve definitive local disease control
4. Demonstrate the relative chemo-responsiveness of a particular cancer or, conversely, chemo-resistance. (Note: Such data can be helpful in the decision as to whether an aggressive and successful attempt to achieve local disease control can realistically also be associated with long-term survival).
5. Help determine the potential clinical utility associated with the continued delivery of *adjuvant chemotherapy* following the surgical removal/primary radiation treatment of all viable local tumor (in the absence of knowledge of the existence of any metastatic disease).
6. Avoid a negative impact on outcome in settings where the performance of definitive surgery/radiation unfortunately must be delayed (for example, due to limited personnel, operating room time/space, or equipment)
7. Obtain tissue prior to and following chemotherapy to determine changes in the molecular profile of residual cancer with the goal that such information may help predict which therapies might be most beneficial to administer.

Table 1. Rationale for neoadjuvant chemotherapy of malignant disease

3. Conclusion

As outlined in this chapter there is a strong rationale for the delivery of systemic therapy prior to definitive local/regional treatment of a malignancy. It is relevant to note that not all of the justifications for this approach highlighted in Table 1 will be operative in a particular clinical setting. Further, it is important to acknowledge the actual benefits associated with this therapeutic approach in specific situations will likely ultimately need to be examined in well-designed evidence-based clinical trials.

However, the genuine opportunity to both increase the patient populations able to undergo definitive local cancer control while at the same time optimizing quality-of-life outcomes that are inherent in the general concept of the neoadjuvant approach should serve as a strong stimulus to encourage clinical investigators to actively address the use of this strategy as an important component of routine cancer management.

Author details

Maurie Markman

Address all correspondence to: maurie.markman@ctca-hope.com

From Cancer Treatment Centers of America, Eastern Regional Medical Center, Philadelphia, PA, USA

References

[1] Arvold, N. D, Ryan, D. P, Niemierko, A, et al. Long-term outcomes of neoadjuvant chemotherapy before chemoradiation for locally advanced pancreatic cancer. Cancer (2012). , 118, 3026-3035.

[2] James, N. D, Hussain, S. A, Hall, E, et al. Radiotherapy with or without chemotherapy in muscle-invasive bladder cancer. N Engl J Med (2012). , 366, 1477-1488.

[3] Van Hagen, P. Hulshof MCCM, van Lanschot JJB, et al. Preoperative chemoradiotherapy for esophageal or junctional cancer. N Engl J Med (2012). , 366, 2074-2084.

[4] Vergote, I, Trope, C. G, Amant, F, et al. Neoadjuvant chemotherapy or primary surgery in stage IIIC or IV ovarian cancer. N Engl J Med (2010). , 363, 943-953.

[5] Wang, J, Estrella, J. S, Peng, L, et al. Histologic tumor involvement of superior mesenteric vein/portal vein predicts poor prognosis with stage II pancreatic adenocarcinoma treated with neoadjuvant chemoradiation. Cancer (2012). , 118, 3801-3811.

[6] Bear, H. D, Tang, G, Rastogi, P, et al. Bevacizumab added to neoadjuvant chemotherapy for breast cancer. N Engl J Med (2012). , 366, 310-320.

[7] Prowell, T. M, & Pazdur, R. Pathological complete response and accelerated drug approval in early breast cancer. N Engl J Med (2012). , 2438-2441.

Chapter 6

Neoadjuvant Chemotherapy for Cervical Cancer: Rationale and Evolving Data

Sung-Jong Lee, Jin-Hwi Kim, Joo-Hee Yoon,
Keun-Ho Lee, Dong-Choon Park, Chan-Joo Kim,
Soo-Young Hur, Tae-Chul Park,
Seog-Nyeon Bae and Jong-Sup Park

Additional information is available at the end of the chapter

http://dx.doi.org/10.5772/53406

1. Introduction

Cervical cancer is still the second most common female malignancy and the second most common cause of cancer-related mortality in women worldwide. [1] In 1999, the National Cancer Institute showed that in addition to radiotherapy, cisplatin chemotherapy produced a therapeutic effect in women with locally advanced cervical cancer (LACC) in 5 randomized trials. [2-7] However, the standard treatments for early cervical cancer have traditionally comprised radical hysterectomy with lymph node dissection or cisplatin-based chemoradiation. [8] Unfortunately, poor prognosis was observed in patients with tumors more than 4 cm in diameter and a poor survival rate of 50–60% was noted in patients with large tumors. To improve the therapeutic results, a new approach with neoadjuvant chemotherapy (NACT) followed by radical surgery or chemoradiation has been introduced. The definition of NACT in cervical cancer is the administration of chemotherapy for the purpose of reducing the cancer volume before the main treatment. In the late 1980s, a pilot study of NACT with cisplatin, bleomycin, and methotrexate performed for 33 patients with a tumor larger than 4 cm showed a response rate of 75.7% (complete response 12.1%, partial response 63.6%) on histologic examination. The sites showing a sensitive response to NACT were the vagina, cervix, and parametrium, in that order. [9] In 1989, Kim et al. performed NACT with vinblastine, bleomycin, and cisplatin (VBP) in 54 patients and reported a high response rate (81.0%), a low incidence of lymph node metastasis (20%), and an improvement in the 2-year tumor free survival rate (94%). [10]

Since 1990, trials evaluating NACT combined with surgery and/or radiation therapy have been undertaken, and this combination therapy has been compared with standard treatments such as radical surgery, radiation therapy, and concurrent chemoradiation.

The aim of this chapter is to investigate the chemotherapy agents used in NACT, know the rationale of NACT before surgery and/or radiation therapy, and review the articles comparing results of NACT with that of surgery or radiation for cervical cancer.

2. Agents used in NACT

Historically, cisplatin has been considered the most active platinum agent drug, with a response rate of 20% in cervical cancer. Although a higher response rate is reported with a dose of 100 mg/m^2 than with a dose of 50 mg/m^2, no differences in complete remission rate, overall survival (OS), and progression-free interval (PFS) were observed between these doses. A high dose of cisplatin was reported to be related to nephrotoxicity and myelosuppression. [11] Moreover, alkylating agent groups also contain an ifosfamide agent, which shows a response rate of 20% at a dose of 1.2 g/m^2 for 5 days in cervical cancer. A higher response rate was noted in patients receiving combination chemotherapy with cisplatin and ifosfamide than in patients receiving cisplatin only (31.1% vs 17.8%, $p = 0.004$). However, no significant difference in OS was found between these groups. [12] Doxorubicin is an anthracycline antibiotic drug that inhibits the process of cancer cell replication by intercalation into DNA. The response rate of cervical cancer to doxorubicin is reported as 20%. The most severe side effect of doxorubicin is cardiotoxicity, which can be fatal. [13] Paclitaxel, which belongs to the taxane group of drugs, stabilizes polymerized microtubules and inhibits cell division. Paclitaxel shows broad-range activity against a number of solid tumors, including epithelial ovarian cancer, lung cancer, and breast cancer. A dose of 170 mg/m^2 is administered intravenously for 24 hours every 3 weeks. The response rate of cervical cancer to paclitaxel is reported to be 17%. According to pharmacological studies, the sequence of administration is very important when paclitaxel is combined with cisplatin for chemotherapy. Administration of cisplatin before paclitaxel generates more severe hematological toxicity (e.g., neutropenia) than administration of paclitaxel before cisplatin. This distinction arises because of the delayed clearance of paclitaxel when paclitaxel is administered after cisplatin. [14]

3. Rationale of NACT

In 1997, Sardi et al. reported the first randomized trial to investigate the role of NACT in 205 stage 1B women with cervical squamous cell carcinoma. [15] The NACT regimen with 10-day intervals included 3 cycles composed of 50 mg/m^2 cisplatin, 1 mg/m^2 vincristine, and 25 mg/m^2 bleomycin. NACT enabled radical hysterectomy for inoperable bulky cervix cancer and improved the rate of complete resectability. [15, 16] NACT reduced the pelvic recurrence rate significantly and increased the survival rate while decreasing the rate of parametrial invasion and lymph node metastasis. An initial tumor size of less than 4.8-cm diameter showed a better response to NACT than a larger tumor size. [16] As the size of the tumor increases, the proportion of hypoxic cancer cells with decreased chemosensitivity increases. Therefore, the potential for complete resection decreases for large tumors. [17, 18] NACT increased the sensitivity of tumor cells to radiation therapy and decreased the proportion of hypoxic cells. Moreover, chemotherapy can be more effectively delivered to tumor volume before blood vessel is destructed by surgery or radiation therapy. [19] However, an undesired delay in the main treatment and resistance to radiation therapy can occur after NACT. [20, 21]

4. Dose of chemotherapy and interval of cycles in NACT

In 2003, the results of a large-scale meta-analysis that systemically reviewed 21 randomized trials were reported. [22] In a comparison of NACT followed by radiation therapy with radiation therapy alone, 2,074 patients in 18 randomized trials were considered for meta-analysis. NACT provided a benefit in survival for cervical cancer patients treated with shorter (interval ≤ 14 days) (hazard Ratio {HR}, 0.83; 95% confidence interval {CI}, 0.69–1.00; $p = 0.046$) and more dose-intensive (cisplatin ≥ 25 mg/ m^2/cycle) (HR, 0.91; 95% CI, 0.78–1.05, $p = 0.20$) regimens. In contrast, survival was less favorable in patients treated with longer (interval ≥ 14 days) (HR, 1.25; 95% CI, 1.07–1.46; $p = 0.005$) and less dose-intensive (cisplatin ≤ 25 mg/m^2/ cycle) (HR, 1.35; 95% CI, 1.11–1.14; $p = 0.002$) regimens. Moreover, in a comparison of NACT followed by surgery with radiation therapy, 872 patients from 5 randomized trials were reviewed and a significant decrease in the risk of death was found (HR, 0.65; 95% CI, 0.53–0.80; $p = 0.0004$). As a result, a short interval and a high dose of cisplatin appear to offer a great advantage for survival in cervical cancer patients. [22]

5. Neoadjuvant chemotherapy plus surgery versus surgery for cervical cancer

In 2010, the Cochrane Database of Systematic Reviews curated by the MRC Clinical Trial Unit, London, UK, [23] demonstrated the role of NACT in women with early or LACC. This systemic review included 1072 patients, and outcomes such as OS, PFS, pathological response, recurrence rate, and resection rates were investigated. Increased PFS (HR, 0.76; 95% CI, 0.62–0.94; $p = 0.01$), decreased rate of parametrial invasion (odds ratio {OR}, 0.58; 95% CI, 0.41–0.82; $p = 0.002$), decreased rate of lymph node metastasis (OR, 0.54; 95% CI, 0.39–0.73; $p < 0.0001$), reduced recurrence at both local (OR, 0.76; 95% CI, 0.49–1.17; $p = 0.21$) and distant (OR, 0.68; 95% CI, 0.41–1.13; $p = 0.13$) sites, and resection rate (OR, 1.55; 95% CI, 0.96–2.50; $p = 0.07$) were observed in this review. Disappointingly, no OS benefit was noted (HR, 0.85; 95% CI, 0.67–1.07; $p = 0.17$). Although favorable results were noted in patients treated with NACT followed by surgery, a significant advantage with regard to OS was not seen. Therefore, the beneficial role of NACT over surgery alone is still unclear in women with early-stage or LACC. [23]

6. Neoadjuvant chemotherapy plus radical surgery versus radiation therapy

Between 1990 and 1996, a randomized trial was performed in 14 Italian centers, and 441 women were categorized into 2 groups: NACT followed by surgery patients and radiation only patients. For patients with stage IB2 to IIB tumors, treatment with NACT and surgery showed a 5-year survival rate of 64.7% and a PFS rate of 59.7%. These values were significantly greater than those in the radiation only group (18.3% and 13.0%, respectively) ($p = 0.005$ and $p = 0.02$, respectively). [24] However, an analysis of patients with stage III tumors only showed no significant differences in OS and PFS (OS: 41.6% vs 36.7%, $p = 0.36$; PFS: 41.9% vs 36.4%, $p = 0.29$). With this result, it may be suggested that the more progressed is tumor volume, the lesser benefit of NACT and subsequent surgery is noted over radiation therapy. Multivariate analysis showed that OS and PFS were significantly affected by stage, treatment modality, cervical tumor diameter, and lymph node metastasis on computed tomography/lymphangiography. The relative risk of OS in patients treated with NACT plus surgery compared with patients treated with radiation only was 0.63 (95% CI, 0.47–0.86). However, no significant differences were observed in the pattern of recurrence between the NACT plus surgery group and the radiation group. [24] In this study, NACT followed by surgery showed better results with regard to OS and PFS than the radiation only group.

On the other hand, Cervical Cancer Study Group of the Asian Oceanian Clinical Oncology Association [25] performed a chemotherapy of cisplatin 60 mg/m^2 and epirubicin 110 mg/m^2 at 3-week intervals for three cycles, and reported that NACT prior to radiation for cervical cancer patients with stage IIB-IVA showed a significantly higher pelvic recurrence rate compared to those who were treated with radiation therapy alone ($p < 0.003$). Also, lower response rate and inferior survival outcome were noted in patients treated with NACT before radiation compared to patients who received radiation therapy alone. This randomized trial of epirubicin and cisplatin chemotherapy followed by pelvic radiation in LACC failed to demonstrate advantage to NACT prior to radiation over radiation therapy alone in local control and tumor response. [25]

7. Neoadjuvant chemotherapy plus radical surgery versus surgery only and concurrent chemoradiation therapy only

Retrospective review of the follow-up reports of 476 patients with stage IB2-IIB cervical cancer enrolled from 2000 to 2005 indicated that patients treated with NACT followed by surgery showed significantly higher 5-year survival rates than both the radical surgery (OS: HR, 1.813; $p = 0.0175$) and concurrent chemoradiation treatment (OS: HR, 3.157; $p < 0.0001$) groups. [26] Moreover, in the NACT plus surgery group, NACT with a combination of paclitaxel and cisplatin (TP) chemotherapy improved the long-term disease-free survival (DFS) and OS compared NACT with a chemotherapy regimen of vincristine, bleomycin, and cisplatin (VBP) ($p < 0.001$). A tumor size of more than 4 cm caused a significant reduction in both the 5-year

DFS and OS rates (HR, 1.762; 95% CI, 1.131–2.744; $p = 0.0122$ and HR, 1.669; 95% CI, 1.164–2.392; $p = 0.0053$, respectively). The limitation of this study is that a selection bias resulted because of the retrospective nature of the investigation. In terms of the proportion of patients with a tumor larger than 4 cm, a higher rate was observed in the concurrent chemoradiotherapy group than in the NACT plus surgery group (77.7% vs 49.7%). [26]

8. The drug combination and regimen of NACT

In 1983, Friedlander reported that a combination of cisplatin (60 mg/m^2 on day 1), vinblastine (4 mg/m^2 on days 1 and 2), and bleomycin (15 mg on days 1, 8, and 15) followed by radiation therapy and/or surgery was performed for 35 cervical cancer patients at 3-week intervals. In this study, 66% of cancer patients showed responsiveness, with 18% showing complete responsiveness, to NACT with radiation and/or surgery. [27]

Between 1983 and 1990, Hwang et al. enrolled 80 women with stage IB to IIB cervical cancer with a tumor diameter of more than 4 cm. A NACT regimen of VBP followed by radical hysterectomy with pelvic lymphadenectomy showed overall 5-year and 10-year DFS rates of 82.0% and 79.4%, respectively. The VBP regimen is considered a tolerable combination with low hematological toxicity and a favorable response rate. [28] In 1990, Lara et al. reported that the administration of cisplatin and ifosfamide chemotherapy was an effective anti-cancer remedy for cervical cancer IIIB patients as a neoadjuvant treatment. The chemotherapy schedule was composed of 20 mg/m^2 cisplatin on days 1–5 and 1.5 g/m^2 ifosfamide on days 1–5. Thereafter, radiotherapy was performed, and 62.5% of patients experienced at least a 50% reduction in tumor size. The authors reported that these results were superior to those for radiotherapy alone. [29]

The SNAP01 (Studio Neo-Adjuvante Portio) randomized trial was performed in 21 Italian centers from 1997 to 2000, and 219 patients were divided into 2 groups: 113 women were treated with the ifosfamide, and cisplatin (IP) combination regimen and 106 received the paclitaxel, ifosfamide, and cisplatin (TIP) combination regimen. [30] The response rate of patients treated with the IP regimen was 23%, whereas that of patients treated with the TIP regimen was 48% ($p = 0.0004$). However, the HR was not significant for patients treated with the TIP regimen (HR, 0.66; 95% CI, 0.39–1.10; $p = 0.11$) and those treated with the IP regimen with respect to OS. Hematological toxicity was more severe in the TIP regimen group; therefore, women older than 70 years or those with renal problems were not recommended for intense NACT. The authors suggested that the optimal response rate could be used as a surrogate marker for survival. Thus, optimal response rate can be used as a cornerstone to quickly monitor the therapeutic results in cervical cancer patients.

Helena et al. [31] performed NACT in 141 women with cervical cancer 1B (1B1: 30 patients, 1B2: 111 patients) from 1998 to 2008. A regimen of cisplatin (75 mg/m^2) and ifosfamide (2 g/m^2) was used in patients with squamous cell cervical cancer and a combination of cisplatin (75 mg/m^2) and doxorubicin (35 mg/m^2) was used in women diagnosed with adenocarcinoma. The NACT cycle was 3 days, and the interval was 10–14 days. The most common hematological toxicity was neutropenia. Interestingly, 69.5% of women who were treated with NACT experienced a reduction in tumor size of more than 50%, and 11.3% of patients showed no residual malignancy on pathological examination after NACT. Further, the 5-year survival rate was 80.6%, and 56.8% of patients are now disease free.

From 1999 to 2004, Bae et al. [32] enrolled 112 patients with stage IB to IIB tumors who were treated with 3 cycles of NACT composed of cisplatin (60 mg/m^2 on days 1 and 2) and etoposide (100 mg/m^2 on day 1). Etoposide is a topoisomerase inhibitor that inhibits the re-ligation of DNA strands and induces breaks in DNA strands. Etoposide can induce cell death through autophagy. The authors demonstrated that NACT followed by surgery resulted in 5-year OS and PFS rates of 88.1% and 60.5%, respectively.

Between 2000 and 2002, Park et al. [19] administered a NACT regimen of paclitaxel (60 mg/m^2 on day 1) and cisplatin (60 mg/m^2 on day 1) for 43 stage IB2 to IIB cervical cancer patients, with 3 cycles every 10 days. The authors reported a high response rate of 90.7%, with a complete response rate of 39.5% (11.6% confirmed by pathology), a partial response rate of 51.2%, and no cases of progression. Thirty-one of 43 patients (72.1%) experienced downstaging of cervical cancer. The 43 patients underwent radical hysterectomy and lymph node dissection after NACT. The 2- and 5-year DFS rates were 94.5% and 89.2%, respectively. Response after NACT, differentiation of cancer cells, and metastasis were reported to be associated with survival. The authors insisted that the reduced delay because of the shorter interval of NACT had a positive effect on survival. [33]

In 2004, NACT was successfully used in fertility-preserving radical trachelectomy for young women with early-stage cervical cancer. The chemotherapy regimen was composed of paclitaxel (175 mg/m^2 on day 1), cisplatin (75 mg/m^2 on day 2), and ifosfamide (5 g/m^2 over 24 hours). [34]

Between January 2006 and December 2009, 123 women with stage IB2 to IIA cervical cancer were randomly divided into 4 groups. The NACT combination was cisplatin (50 mg/m^2) and 5-fluorouracil (750 mg/m^2) at a 2-week interval. No significant differences in 3-year PFS and OS were observed between the 4 groups. [35]

Between 2007 and 2010, 46 cancer patients with stage IB2 to IIIB tumors were enrolled. The NACT schedule was topotecan (0.75 mg/m^2 on days 1–3) followed by cisplatin (75 mg/m^2 on day 1). The authors examined the therapeutic results in patients treated with NACT followed by surgery. They found that 89.5% of patients experienced a pathological response and 15.8% achieved a complete response. The 2-year PFS and OS of the 38 patients treated with NACT and surgery were 79% and 95%, respectively. [36]

In 2012, the Japanese Gynecologic Oncology Group reported a phase II NACT study with irinotecan hydrochloride and nedaplatin followed by radical hysterectomy for bulky stage IB2 to IIB cervical squamous cell carcinoma. Sixty-six patients were treated with irinotecan (60 mg/m^2 on days 1 and 8) and nedaplatin (80 mg/m^2 on day 1) with a 21-day interval. Radical hysterectomy was performed after NACT, and the response rate was 75.8%. Of these patients, 72.2% complained of neutropenia, and the side effects of NACT were acceptable. [37]

9. Neoadjuvant chemotherapy plus radical surgery followed by chemotherapy

Between 2000 and 2007, NACT (cisplatin 100 mg/m^2 and paclitaxel 175 mg/m^2, 3 cycles every 3 weeks) plus surgery followed by 4 cycles of platinum-based adjuvant chemotherapy was performed by Angioli et al. The authors reported that the 5-year OS and DFS rates were 81% and 70%, respectively. The 5-year OS rates of cervical cancer patients with positive and negative lymph nodes were 75% and 88%, respectively. The authors showed that adjuvant chemotherapy after NACT and surgery could be useful for patients with LACC. [38]

10. Currently ongoing randomized trial

A randomized phase III trial comparing the effectiveness of cisplatin-based NACT followed by radical hysterectomy with the effectiveness of concomitant radiotherapy and chemotherapy in patients with stage IB2 or stage II cervical cancer has been undertaken by the European Organization for Research and Treatment of Cancer (55994). However, the results of that phase III trial have been not yet published.

11. Conclusion

A review of the literature associated with NACT showed that most chemotherapy regimens included cisplatin (Table 1 and Table 2). Recently, the number of clinical trials that include the use of paclitaxel chemotherapy has gradually increased. A short interval between cycles and a high dose of cisplatin were considered optimal for NACT. Three cycles was the most frequently used method in NACT for cervical cancer. In general, the side effects and toxicity of NACT seemed acceptable for patients with cervical cancer. In a review of medical literatures, high response rate after cisplatin-based NACT provided an advantage to surgery and prevention of lymph node metastasis. Moreover, NACT prior to surgery showed acceptable improvement in survival rate in phase III trial. However, no definitive agreement on the best management strategy for NACT has been determined for early and LACC. Therefore, clinicians should carefully compare the efficacy of NACT with the disadvantages of the delayed start of the main treatment and the toxicities associated with chemotherapy.

In the future, early markers or clinical variables for monitoring the effect of NACT during the early phase may be helpful for determining the optimal treatment for cervical cancer patients. Further, drugs that are highly effective for cervical cancer will need to be developed for the NACT regimen. For the determination of optimal treatment in cervical cancer, advantages of NACT should be evaluated in phase III trial compared to standard treatments.

Authors	Publication	Number	Stage	Comparison	Response rate
Friedlander [27]	1983	35	IIB	cisplatin (60 mg/m^2 day1), vinblastine (4 mg/m^2, days 1 and 2), and bleomycin (15 mg, days 1, 8, and 15) followed by radiation therapy and/or surgery	66% (complete response 18%)
Lara [29]	1990	26	IIIB	cisplatin (20 mg/m^2 on day 1-5) and ifosfamide (1.5 g/ m^2 on day 1-5)	62.5%
Hwang [28]	2001	80	IB-IIB	cisplatin (50 mg/m^2 day1), vinblastine (4 mg/ m^2, days 1), and bleomycin (16 mg/ m^2, days1, 2)	93.7% (complete response 50%)
Park [19]	2004	43	IB-IIB	paclitaxel (60 mg/m^2, day 1) and cisplatin (60 mg/m^2, day 1)	90.7%
Buda [30]	2005	113	IB-IV	cisplatin 75 mg/m^2 paclitaxel 175 mg/m2 ifosfamide 5 g/m2	48%
Bae [32]	2008	112	IB-IIB	cisplatin (60 mg/m^2, days 1, 2) and etoposide (100 mg/m^2, day 1)	69.7%
Helena [31]	2010	141	IB	cisplatin (75 mg/m^2) and ifosfamide (2 g/m^2)	69.5%

Table 1. Pilot study of neoadjuvant chemotherapy for cervical cancer

Authors	Publication	Number	Stage	Comparison	Neoadjuvant chemotherapy
Souhami [39]	1991	107	IIIB	NACT+RT vs RT	Bleomycin 15U IM days 1-4, vincristine 1mg/m^2 day 1, mitomycin C 10 mg/m^2 day 1, cisplatin 50 mg/m^2 day 1,
Chauvergne [40]	1993	151	IIB~III	NACT+RT vs RT	methotrexate, chlorambucil, vincristine, cisplatin
Tattersall [25]	1995	260	IIB~IVA	NACT+RT vs RT	cisplatin 60 mg/m^2 and epirubicin 110 mg/m^2 day 1
Sardi [15]	1997	205	IB	NACT+RT vs RT	vincristine 1mg/m^2 day 1, cisplatin 50 mg/m^2 day 1, bleomycin 25 mg/m^2 days 1-3
Kumar [41]	1998	184	IIB~IVA	NACT+RT vs RT	bleomycin, ifosfamide, cisplatin
Symonds [42]	2000	204	IIB~IVA	NACT+RT vs RT	methotrexate 100 mg/m^2, cisplatin 50 mg/m^2
Chang [43]	2000	124	IB~IIA	NACT+RS vs RT	vincristine 1mg/m^2 day 1, cisplatin 50 mg/m^2 day 1, bleomycin 25 mg/m^2 days 1-3
Herod [44]	2000	172	IB~IVA	NACT+RS vs RT	bleomycin 30 units/24-hour infusion, ifosfamide 5 g/m^2/24 hours, cisplatin 50 mg/m^2
Benedetti-Panici [24]	2002	441	IB~III	NACT+RS vs RT	cisplatin-based NACT (with a "/>240 mg/m^2 total cisplatin dose)
Wen [35]	2012	123	IB-IIA	NACT+RS vs RS vs BT +RS vs IACT	cisplatin (50 mg/m^2) and 5-fluorouracil (750 mg/m^2) at a 2-week interval

NACT:neoadjuvant chemotherapy, RS: radical surgery, RT: radiation therapy, BT:Brachy radiation, IACT:Intra-arterial chemotherapy

Table 2. Randomized controlled trial about neoadjuvant chemotherapy for cervical cancer

Author details

Sung-Jong Lee, Jin-Hwi Kim, Joo-Hee Yoon, Keun-Ho Lee, Dong-Choon Park, Chan-Joo Kim, Soo-Young Hur, Tae-Chul Park, Seog-Nyeon Bae and Jong-Sup Park

Department of Obstetrics and Gynecology, College of Medicine, The Catholic University of Korea, Seoul, Korea

References

[1] Parkin, D. M, Pisani, P, & Ferlay, J. Estimates of the worldwide incidence of eighteen major cancers in 1985. Int J Cancer (1993). , 54(4), 594-606.

[2] Whitney, C. W, Sause, W, Bundy, B. N, Malfetano, J. H, Hannigan, E. V, Fowler, W. C, et al. Randomized comparison of fluorouracil plus cisplatin versus hydroxyurea as an adjunct to radiation therapy in stage IIB-IVA carcinoma of the cervix with negative para-aortic lymph nodes: a Gynecologic Oncology Group and Southwest Oncology Group study. J Clin Oncol (1999). , 17(5), 1339-48.

[3] Morris, M, Eifel, P. J, Lu, J, Grigsby, P. W, Levenback, C, Stevens, R. E, et al. Pelvic radiation with concurrent chemotherapy compared with pelvic and para-aortic radiation for high-risk cervical cancer. N Engl J Med (1999). , 340(15), 1137-43.

[4] Rose, P. G, Bundy, B. N, Watkins, E. B, Thigpen, J. T, Deppe, G, Maiman, M. A, et al. Concurrent cisplatin-based radiotherapy and chemotherapy for locally advanced cervical cancer. N Engl J Med (1999). , 340(15), 1144-53.

[5] Keys, H. M, Bundy, B. N, Stehman, F. B, Muderspach, L. I, Chafe, W. E, Suggs, C. L, et al. Cisplatin, radiation, and adjuvant hysterectomy compared with radiation and adjuvant hysterectomy for bulky stage IB cervical carcinoma. N Engl J Med (1999). , 340(15), 1154-61.

[6] Peters, W. A. rd, Liu PY, Barrett RJ, 2nd, Stock RJ, Monk BJ, Berek JS, et al. Concurrent chemotherapy and pelvic radiation therapy compared with pelvic radiation therapy alone as adjuvant therapy after radical surgery in high-risk early-stage cancer of the cervix. J Clin Oncol (2000). , 18(8), 1606-13.

[7] Thomas, G. M. Improved treatment for cervical cancer--concurrent chemotherapy and radiotherapy. N Engl J Med (1999). , 340(15), 1198-200.

[8] Benedet, J. L, Odicino, F, Maisonneuve, P, Beller, U, Creasman, W. T, Heintz, A. P, et al. Carcinoma of the cervix uteri. J Epidemiol Biostat (2001). , 6(1), 7-43.

[9] Benedetti Panici PScambia G, Greggi S, Di Roberto P, Baiocchi G, Mancuso S. Neoadjuvant chemotherapy and radical surgery in locally advanced cervical carcinoma: a pilot study. Obstet Gynecol (1988). Pt 1): 344-8.

[10] Kim, D. S, Moon, H, Kim, K. T, Hwang, Y. Y, Cho, S. H, & Kim, S. R. Two-year survival: preoperative adjuvant chemotherapy in the treatment of cervical cancer stages Ib and II with bulky tumor. Gynecol Oncol (1989). , 33(2), 225-30.

[11] Bonomi, P, Blessing, J. A, & Stehman, F. B. DiSaia PJ, Walton L, Major FJ. Randomized trial of three cisplatin dose schedules in squamous-cell carcinoma of the cervix: a Gynecologic Oncology Group study. J Clin Oncol (1985). , 3(8), 1079-85.

[12] Omura, G. A, Blessing, J. A, Vaccarello, L, Berman, M. L, Clarke-pearson, D. L, Mutch, D. G, et al. Randomized trial of cisplatin versus cisplatin plus mitolactol versus cisplatin plus ifosfamide in advanced squamous carcinoma of the cervix: a Gynecologic Oncology Group study. J Clin Oncol (1997). , 15(1), 165-71.

[13] Wallace, H. J. Jr., Hreshchyshyn MM, Wilbanks GD, Boronow RC, Fowler WC, Jr., Blessing JA. Comparison of the therapeutic effects of adriamycin alone versus adriamycin plus vincristine versus adriamycin plus cyclophosphamide in the treatment of advanced carcinoma of the cervix. Cancer Treat Rep (1978). , 62(10), 1435-41.

[14] Mcguire, W. P, Blessing, J. A, Moore, D, Lentz, S. S, & Photopulos, G. Paclitaxel has moderate activity in squamous cervix cancer. A Gynecologic Oncology Group study. J Clin Oncol (1996). , 14(3), 792-5.

[15] Sardi, J. E, Giaroli, A, Sananes, C, Ferreira, M, Soderini, A, Bermudez, A, et al. Long-term follow-up of the first randomized trial using neoadjuvant chemotherapy in stage Ib squamous carcinoma of the cervix: the final results. Gynecol Oncol (1997). , 67(1), 61-9.

[16] Sardi, J, Sananes, C, Giaroli, A, & Maya, G. di Paola G. Neoadjuvant chemotherapy in locally advanced carcinoma of the cervix uteri. Gynecol Oncol (1990). , 38(3), 486-93.

[17] Benedetti-panici, P, Greggi, S, Scambia, G, Amoroso, M, Salerno, M. G, Maneschi, F, et al. Long-term survival following neoadjuvant chemotherapy and radical surgery in locally advanced cervical cancer. Eur J Cancer (1998). , 34(3), 341-6.

[18] Sananes, C, Giaroli, A, Soderini, A, Guardado, N, Snaidas, L, Bermudez, A, et al. Neoadjuvant chemotherapy followed by radical hysterectomy and postoperative adjuvant chemotherapy in the treatment of carcinoma of the cervix uteri: long-term follow-up of a pilot study. Eur J Gynaecol Oncol (1998). , 19(4), 368-73.

[19] Park, D. C, Kim, J. H, Lew, Y. O, Kim, D. H, & Namkoong, S. E. Phase II trial of neoadjuvant paclitaxel and cisplatin in uterine cervical cancer. Gynecol Oncol (2004). , 92(1), 59-63.

[20] Gonzalez-martin, A, Gonzalez-cortijo, L, Carballo, N, Garcia, J. F, Lapuente, F, Rojo, A, et al. The current role of neoadjuvant chemotherapy in the management of cervical carcinoma. Gynecol Oncol (2008). Suppl 2): S, 36-40.

[21] Rowinsky, E. K, Gilbert, M. R, Mcguire, W. P, Noe, D. A, Grochow, L. B, Forastiere, A. A, et al. Sequences of taxol and cisplatin: a phase I and pharmacologic study. J Clin Oncol (1991). , 9(9), 1692-703.

[22] Neoadjuvant chemotherapy for locally advanced cervical cancer: a systematic review and meta-analysis of individual patient data from 21 randomised trialsEur J Cancer (2003). , 39(17), 2470-86.

[23] Rydzewska, L, Tierney, J, Vale, C. L, & Symonds, P. R. Neoadjuvant chemotherapy plus surgery versus surgery for cervical cancer. Cochrane Database Syst Rev (2010). CD007406.

[24] Benedetti-panici, P, Greggi, S, Colombo, A, Amoroso, M, Smaniotto, D, Giannarelli, D, et al. Neoadjuvant chemotherapy and radical surgery versus exclusive radiotherapy in locally advanced squamous cell cervical cancer: results from the Italian multicenter randomized study. J Clin Oncol (2002). , 20(1), 179-88.

[25] Tattersall, M. H, Lorvidhaya, V, Vootiprux, V, Cheirsilpa, A, Wong, F, Azhar, T, et al. Randomized trial of epirubicin and cisplatin chemotherapy followed by pelvic radiation in locally advanced cervical cancer. Cervical Cancer Study Group of the Asian Oceanian Clinical Oncology Association. J Clin Oncol (1995). , 13(2), 444-51.

[26] Yin, M, Zhao, F, Lou, G, Zhang, H, Sun, M, Li, C, et al. The long-term efficacy of neoadjuvant chemotherapy followed by radical hysterectomy compared with radical surgery alone or concurrent chemoradiotherapy on locally advanced-stage cervical cancer. Int J Gynecol Cancer (2011). , 21(1), 92-9.

[27] Friedlander, M, Kaye, S. B, Sullivan, A, Atkinson, K, Elliott, P, Coppleson, M, et al. Cervical carcinoma: a drug-responsive tumor--experience with combined cisplatin, vinblastine, and bleomycin therapy. Gynecol Oncol (1983). , 16(2), 275-81.

[28] Hwang, Y. Y, Moon, H, Cho, S. H, Kim, K. T, Moon, Y. J, Kim, S. R, et al. Ten-year survival of patients with locally advanced, stage ib-iib cervical cancer after neoadjuvant chemotherapy and radical hysterectomy. Gynecol Oncol (2001). , 82(1), 88-93.

[29] Lara, P. C, Garcia-puche, J. L, & Pedraza, V. Cisplatin-ifosfamide as neoadjuvant chemotherapy in stage IIIB cervical uterine squamous-cell carcinoma. Cancer Chemother Pharmacol (1990). Suppl: S, 36-8.

[30] Buda, A, Fossati, R, Colombo, N, Fei, F, & Floriani, I. Gueli Alletti D, et al. Randomized trial of neoadjuvant chemotherapy comparing paclitaxel, ifosfamide, and cisplatin with ifosfamide and cisplatin followed by radical surgery in patients with locally advanced squamous cell cervical carcinoma: the SNAP01 (Studio Neo-Adjuvante Portio) Italian Collaborative Study. J Clin Oncol (2005). , 23(18), 4137-45.

[31] Robova, H, Halaska, M, Pluta, M, Skapa, P, Strnad, P, Lisy, J, et al. The role of neoadjuvant chemotherapy and surgery in cervical cancer. Int J Gynecol Cancer (2010). Suppl 2): S, 42-6.

[32] Bae, J. H, Lee, S. J, Lee, A, Park, Y. G, Bae, S. N, Park, J. S, et al. Neoadjuvant cisplatin and etoposide followed by radical hysterectomy for stage 1B-2B cervical cancer. Gynecol Oncol (2008). , 111(3), 444-8.

[33] Park, D. C, Suh, M. J, & Yeo, S. G. Neoadjuvant paclitaxel and cisplatin in uterine cervical cancer: long-term results. Int J Gynecol Cancer (2009). , 19(5), 943-7.

[34] Plante, M, Lau, S, Brydon, L, & Swenerton, K. LeBlanc R, Roy M. Neoadjuvant chemotherapy followed by vaginal radical trachelectomy in bulky stage IB1 cervical cancer: case report. Gynecol Oncol (2006). , 101(2), 367-70.

[35] Wen, H, Wu, X, Li, Z, Wang, H, Zang, R, Sun, M, et al. A prospective randomized controlled study on multiple neoadjuvant treatments for patients with stage IB2 to IIA cervical cancer. Int J Gynecol Cancer (2012). , 22(2), 296-302.

[36] Manci, N, & Marchetti, C. Di Tucci C, Giorgini M, Esposito F, Palaia I, et al. A prospective phase II study of topotecan (Hycamtin(R)) and cisplatin as neoadjuvant chemotherapy in locally advanced cervical cancer. Gynecol Oncol (2011). , 122(2), 285-90.

[37] Yamaguchi, S, Nishimura, R, Yaegashi, N, Kiguchi, K, Sugiyama, T, Kita, T, et al. Phase II study of neoadjuvant chemotherapy with irinotecan hydrochloride and nedaplatin followed by radical hysterectomy for bulky stage Ib2 to IIb, cervical squamous cell carcinoma: Japanese Gynecologic Oncology Group study (JGOG 1065). Oncol Rep (2012). , 28(2), 487-93.

[38] Angioli, R, Plotti, F, Montera, R, Aloisi, A, Luvero, D, Capriglione, S, et al. Neoadjuvant chemotherapy plus radical surgery followed by chemotherapy in locally advanced cervical cancer. Gynecol Oncol (2012).

[39] Souhami, L, Gil, R. A, Allan, S. E, Canary, P. C, Araujo, C. M, Pinto, L. H, et al. A randomized trial of chemotherapy followed by pelvic radiation therapy in stage IIIB carcinoma of the cervix. J Clin Oncol (1991). , 9(6), 970-7.

[40] Chauvergne, J, Lhomme, C, Rohart, J, Heron, J. F, Ayme, Y, Goupil, A, et al. Neoadjuvant chemotherapy of stage IIb or III cancers of the uterine cervix. Long-term results of a multicenter randomized trial of 151 patients]. Bull Cancer (1993). , 80(12), 1069-79.

[41] Kumar, L, Grover, R, Pokharel, Y. H, Chander, S, Kumar, S, Singh, R, et al. Neoadjuvant chemotherapy in locally advanced cervical cancer: two randomised studies. Aust N Z J Med (1998). , 28(3), 387-90.

[42] Symonds, R. P, Habeshaw, T, Reed, N. S, Paul, J, Pyper, E, Yosef, H, et al. The Scottish and Manchester randomised trial of neo-adjuvant chemotherapy for advanced cervical cancer. Eur J Cancer (2000). , 36(8), 994-1001.

[43] Chang, T. C, Lai, C. H, Hong, J. H, Hsueh, S, Huang, K. G, Chou, H. H, et al. Randomized trial of neoadjuvant cisplatin, vincristine, bleomycin, and radical hysterectomy versus radiation therapy for bulky stage IB and IIA cervical cancer. J Clin Oncol (2000). , 18(8), 1740-7.

[44] Herod, J, Burton, A, Buxton, J, Tobias, J, Luesley, D, Jordan, S, et al. A randomised, prospective, phase III clinical trial of primary bleomycin, ifosfamide and cisplatin (BIP) chemotherapy followed by radiotherapy versus radiotherapy alone in inoperable cancer of the cervix. Ann Oncol (2000). , 11(9), 1175-81.

Chapter 7

Neoadjuvant Chemotherapy in the Management of Advanced Ovarian Cancer and Primary Cancer of the Peritoneum: Rationale and Results

Maurie Markman

Additional information is available at the end of the chapter

http://dx.doi.org/10.5772/55394

1. Introduction

For more than 40 years the standard-of-care in the management of advanced ovarian cancer and primary peritoneal cancer has been an attempt to optimally cytoreduce ("debulk") disease present within abdominal cavity *prior to the administration of cytotoxic chemotherapy* [1-3]. Several justifications have been advanced in support of this general approach to disease management (briefly summarized in Table 1).

Remove all or most macroscopic tumor to permit the subsequent delivery (via capillary flow or intraperitoneal drug delivery) of optimal concentrations to any residual cancer of an effective anti-neoplastic chemotherapy regimen (platinum-based)
Reduce the risk for the development of resistance resulting from the delivery of inadequate concentrations of cytotoxic drug therapy
Rapidly decrease cancer-related symptoms due to the presence of intra-abdominal cancer (e.g., pain, inability to eat)
Enhance the nutritional status to permit improved tolerance of the chemotherapy regimen
Optimize the functional status of the immune system following removal of large tumor bulk

Table 1. Rationale for primary surgical cytoreduction in advanced ovarian cancer

A rather substantial number of single investigators, single institutions, and multi-institutional experiences have reported data that support the concept that patients who undergo successful primary surgery experience an anticipated statistically-significant superior survival outcome compared to patients who are treated with primary chemotherapy (no attempt to cytoreduce the cancer following the diagnosis) or who fail to be able to undergo successful cytoreduction despite a reasonable attempt by a gynecologic cancer surgeon [2-4]. Unfortunately, and rather remarkably considering the extensive use of this strategy, the *utility of primary surgical cytoreduction has never actually been documented in a prospective phase 3 randomized trial.*

In fact, while there should be no legitimate disagreement with the statement that the population of advanced epithelial ovarian cancer patients who initiate platinum-based chemotherapy with the smallest volume of residual cancer will be anticipated to experience the most favorable survival outcome, it remains uncertain today if the "favorable outcome" results from the skills of the individual gynecologic cancer surgeon or is more related to the "favorable biology" of the cancer which also grows and progresses in a pattern and location that is more conducive for resection, in contrast to more aggressive and widespread malignancies. For example, it is quite plausible that the same poorly understood biological/molecular factors that render a particular tumor more chemo-resistant (either *de novo* or early in the clinical course) also substantially influence resectability (e.g., presence or absence of diffuse carcinomatosis within the peritoneal cavity or extensive retroperitoneal involvement with the cancer).

2. Evidence-based data supporting a role for surgical cytoreduction in advanced ovarian cancer at some point during the course of the illness

Despite the absence of phase 3 randomized trial data demonstrating the utility of *primary surgical cytoreduction* in advanced ovarian cancer, a landmark European phase 3 study revealed the benefits of an interval surgical cytoreductive procedure following an initial surgery and the administration of several cycles of cytotoxic chemotherapy [5]. In this trial patients were randomized to undergo primary surgical cytoreduction followed by six cycles of platinum-based chemotherapy versus having the surgery, followed by three cycles of the same chemotherapy, which was followed by a second attempt at surgical cytoreduction ("interval cytoreduction") and then three more cycles of chemotherapy. Patients randomized to the interval surgical procedure experienced a statistically significant improvement in overall survival compared to women not offered this second surgical procedure.

However, a second study conducted in the United States which employed a similar "interval cytoreduction" approach but utilized a cisplatin plus paclitaxel regimen versus cisplatin plus cyclophosphamide utilized in the European study failed to demonstrate an improvement in survival associated with the second surgery [6]. While it is always difficult to compare the outcome results across two independent clinical trials, the difference in the overall aggressiveness of the primary surgical approach in the United States may explain (at least in part) the somewhat surprising differences between the two studies.

Considering the results of these two well-performed evidence-based studies one might suggest the data support the concept that ovarian cancer patients appear to experience benefit from an attempt to maximally cytoreduce intraperitoneal disease but it does not make a major differ-

http://dx.doi.org/10.5772/55394

ence if that surgery is performed at the initial diagnosis or as a component of an attempt to administer primary chemotherapy followed by definitive surgery.

3. Neoadjuvant chemotherapy of advanced ovarian cancer

The rational supporting the use of neoadjuvant chemotherapy in the management of advanced ovarian cancer is outlined in Table 2. The earliest experience with this approach focused on patients who were simply too ill to undergo primary surgery, or were believed to be an unacceptable surgical risk (e.g., large bilateral cancer-related pleural effusions) [7].

Manage patients unable to undergo primary surgical cytoreduction either because of extensive disease or the existence of co-morbidities increasing the risk associated with the procedure
Reduce the morbidity and possibly mortality associated with aggressive surgery of extensive intra-peritoneal ovarian cancer
Improve the nutritional status of patients prior to the performance of a major abdominal surgery, specifically to reduce the risk of a serious adverse event.
Determine if an individual cancer is chemo-sensitive and whether it is appropriate to attempt to cytoreduce the cancer. (The basic argument here is that patients with chemo-resistant cancers are most unlikely to benefit from an attempt at surgical cytoreduction. Of course, surgery may be clinically indicated to provide short-term palliation of distressing cancer-related symptoms [e.g., colostomy for large-bowel obstruction].)

Table 2. Rationale for neoadjuvant chemotherapy of advanced ovarian cancer

However, many patients who achieved a major objective and subjective response following several cycles of platinum-based chemotherapy were found to have sufficiently improved their overall performance status to permit surgical intervention. In several reports documenting the outcome of patients managed in this manner there was evidence that the survival outcomes were not terribly different "compared to" individuals of a similar age and initial tumor volume who were managed with primary surgery followed by chemotherapy [8-10]. It is critical to acknowledge here that such comparisons are fraught with great danger due to the potential for major selection bias in the populations of individuals who might undergo neoadjuvant chemotherapy versus primary surgical cytoreduction [7].

4. Phase 3 trial of primary surgical cytoreduction compared to neoadjuvant chemotherapy followed by surgical cytoreduction in advanced ovarian cancer

In fact, the only way to directly address the issue of the overall clinical utility of primary surgical cytoreduction versus neoadjuvant chemotherapy and a subsequent attempt to achieve maximal surgical cytoreduction would be to perform a randomized trial. In another landmark clinical study a multi-institutional cooperative group consortium reported the results of a well-designed and conducted phase 3 trial involving 670 women with advanced ovarian cancer or primary peritoneal cancer who either underwent primary surgery followed by chemotherapy with carboplatin plus paclitaxel or were treated initially (after the diagnosis was confirmed) with the same chemotherapy followed by cytoreductive surgery with additional chemotherapy subsequently administered [11].

The study outcomes are summarized in Table 3. There was no difference in survival between the two approaches, but overall serious morbidity was considerably lower in the neoadjuvant chemotherapy group. Of interest, within each country where this study was conducted it was observed that compared to the percentage of patients able to be optimally cytoreduced in the primary setting there was a higher proportion of women able to achieve this clinical state in the trial arm where neoadjuvant chemotherapy was followed by interval cytoreduction.

	Primary Surgical Cytoreduction	**Neoadjuvant Chemotherapy**	
Progression-Free Survival (median)	12 months	12 months	Hazard ratio: 1.01
Overall Survival (median)	29 months	30 months	Hazard ratio: 0.98
Mortality (death within 28 days after surgery)	2.5%	0.7%	
Grade 3-4 hemorrhage	7.4%	4.1%	
Infection	8.1%	1.7%	
Venous complications	2.6%	0%	

Table 3. Summary of results of the phase 3 trial comparing primary cytoreductive surgery to neoadjuvant chemotherapy followed by surgery in advanced ovarian cancer [11]

5. Summary and reasonable conclusions regarding utility of neoadjuvant chemotherapy of advanced ovarian cancer based on available evidence-based data

Despite the results of this well-conducted multi-center phase 3 randomized trial there continues to be considerable controversy within the gynecologic cancer clinical research community regarding a standard/routine role for neoadjuvant chemotherapy in the management of advanced ovarian and primary peritoneal cancers. This response should not be surprising when one considers both the number of years primary surgical cytoreductive procedures have been the standard-of-care and the number of trainees worldwide who have been taught this should be the standard.

In fact, some have argued (in the absence of any randomized trial data) for essentially the *opposite approach* in patients with the most advanced disease and have advocated for even more aggressive primary surgery (including resection of metastatic cancer in the liver and chest) rather than chemotherapy followed by surgery after a favorable response is documented [12]. The justification for this strategy is once again retrospective data demonstrating patients with the smallest volume of residual cancer (microscopic disease only) have the most favorable outcomes.

As previously noted, the problem with this conclusion is that it remains completely unknown if such outcomes are the result of the impressive skills of individual surgeons (and those of the institutions caring for patients undergoing such surgery) or simply the selection of patients with the most favorable tumor biology. Of course, it is possible that the true answer to this important question is a variable combination of both factors.

However, despite statements by some in the gynecologic oncology community to the contrary, the current evidence from the conduct of two well-designed and conducted phase 3 randomized trials strongly indicates that acceptable initial management of advanced ovarian cancer includes the delivery of neoadjuvant platinum-based chemotherapy (following the diagnosis of a malignancy consistent with ovarian cancer) and the subsequent performance of an interval cytoreductive procedure designed to remove all residual macroscopic cancer (if technically feasible). This surgery will then be followed by additional chemotherapy designed to optimize both the extent and duration of the response and overall survival.

Author details

Maurie Markman*

Address all correspondence to: maurie.markman@ctca-hope.com

From Cancer Treatment Centers of America, Eastern Regional Medical Center, Philadelphia, PA, USA

References

[1] Hennessy, B. T, Coleman, R. L, & Markman, M. Ovarian Cancer (2009). , 374, 1371-1382.

[2] Markman, M. Concept of optimal surgical cytoreduction in advanced ovarian cancer: A brief critique and a call for action. J Clin Oncol (2007). , 25, 4168-4170.

[3] Griffin, T. Surgical resection of tumor bulk in the primary treatment of ovarian carcinoma. Natl Cancer Inst Monogr (1975). , 42, 101-104.

[4] Bristow, R. E, Tomacruz, R. S, Armstrong, D. K, et al. Survival effect of maximal cytoreductive surgery for advanced ovarian carcinoma during the platinum era: A meta-analysis. J Clin Onocl (2002). , 20, 1248-1259.

[5] Van Der Burg, M. E, Van Lent, M, Buyse, M, et al. The effect of debulking surgery after induction chemotherapy on the prognosis in advanced epithelial ovarian cancer. N Engl J Med (1995). , 332, 629-634.

[6] Rose, P. G, Nerenstone, S, Brady, M. F, et al. Secondary surgical cytoreduction for advanced ovarian carcinoma. N Engl J Med (2004). , 351, 2489-2497.

[7] Bristow, R. E, & Chi, D. S. Platinum-based neoadjuvant chemotherapy and interval surgical cytoreduction for advanced ovarian cancer: A meta-analysis. Gynecol Oncol (2006). , 103, 1070-1076.

[8] Schwartz, P. E, Rutherford, T. J, Chambers, J. T, et al. Neoadjuvant chemotherapy for advanced ovarian cancer: Long-term survival. Gynecologic Oncol (1999). , 72, 93-99.

[9] Surwit, E, Childers, J, Atlas, I, et al. Neoadjuavnt chemotherapy for advanced ovarian cancer. Int J Gynecol Cancer (1996). , 6, 356-361.

[10] Vergote I De Wever ITjalma W, et al. Neoadjuvant chemotherapy or primary debulking surgery in advanced ovarian carcinoma: A retrospective analysis of 285 patients. Gynecol Oncol (1998). , 71, 431-436.

[11] Vergote, I, Trope, C. G, Amant, F, et al. Neoadjuvant chemotherapy or primary surgery in stage IIIC or IV ovarian cancer. N Engl J Med (2010). , 363, 843-953.

[12] Chi, D. S, Eisenhauer, E. L, Zivanovic, O, et al. Improved progression-free and overall survival in advanced ovarian cancer as a result of a change in surgical paradigm. Gynecologic Oncol (2009). , 114, 26-31.